Bypass the Bypass

Restore Circulation Without Surgery

David Rowland

BALBOA.
PRESS

A DIVISION OF HAY HOUSE

Balboa Press books may be ordered through booksellers or by contacting:

Balboa Press
A Division of Hay House
1663 Liberty Drive
Bloomington, IN 47403
www.balboapress.com
1 (877) 407-4847

Print information available on the last page.

ISBN: 978-1-5043-6227-6 (sc)
ISBN: 978-1-5043-6228-3 (e)

Balboa Press rev. date: 08/11/2016

Foreword

The majority of all heart attacks are silent. There is no warning. Unfortunately, the first symptom for many people is death.

Here are some of the most important breakthroughs in medical science in the last decade: inflammation and oxidative stress, *not* cholesterol, causes heart disease. The first detectable signs of occluding arteries are *not* fatty streaks. Bypass surgery does *not* extend lives.

What is irrefutable is that the body has an incredible, innate ability to heal itself, provided we give it both the raw materials and the conditions it needs to do so. When we expose ourselves to hazards (poor nutrition, excessive stress, lack of sleep, etc.) at a rate that exceeds our natural ability to manage these health hazards and we don't give our body enough of the vital raw materials required to fortify these self-repairing systems, then disease manifests.

It was during my graduate program in natural medicine that I came across the first edition of **The Nutritional Bypass: Reverse Atherosclerosis Without Surgery**. This was an eye-opener and a game changer for me. It further substantiated what I was coming to learn over the next four years - that food has a profound impact on our health. Not simply that we can prevent disease, but that we can reverse disease and pathology using the power of nutrition.

Optimal nutrition is irrefutably the cornerstone of good health. The idea is as old as time. You have seen or at the very least heard Hippocrates' famous quote: *"Let food be thy medicine and medicine be thy food"*.

The very popular phrase, "you are what you eat", was first coined in the 1920s by nutritionist Victor Lindlahr, who was a strong believer in the idea that food controls health. *"Ninety per cent of the diseases known to man are caused by cheap foodstuffs. You are what you eat."* wrote Lindlahr. This view has gained many adherents in the last century. But to this very day across North America - where the pharmaceutical industry maintains its control - many conventionally trained doctors are dismissive of nutritional therapies.

Can an optimal diet prevent heart disease? Can certain nutrients stop and even reverse heart disease? Are doctors ready to think outside the pillbox and go beyond cholesterol lowering statins and blood pressure drugs? Conventional practitioners who are dismissive of the power of food and nutrients in health and disease, simply put, have their heads buried in the sand.

It is nearly impossible to ignore powerful scientific studies, such as the Mediterranean diet shown to reduce the incidence of major cardiovascular events by 30 percent. But with all the evidence, a significant nutrition gap remains in North America - a serious disconnect between how patients and doctors perceive diet. From fad diets to unsubstantiated supplements there are so many nutritional therapies out there, so many programs with so many claims, and so little science to back them up that it's no wonder it's hard for sound nutritional therapies to break through.

That is...until now! David Rowland has done it again.

David Rowland is the foremost expert in holistic nutrition, author of 12 highly acclaimed health publications, innovator and publisher of Nutritiapedia®, creator of Nutri-Body® Analysis, founder of The Canadian Nutrition Institute and the Edison Institute of Nutrition. Rowland has cut through the noise and offers no-nonsense nutritional solutions in this most recent edition, ***BYPASS the BYPASS: Restore Circulation Without Surgery.*** This book is the most relevant, useful and comprehensive guide to contemporary holistic nutrition for reversing heart disease.

If heart disease runs in your family, if you have a known personal risk of heart disease, or if you're just very smart to be proactive and not fall victim to heart disease, the arterial cleansing program you'll learn about in these pages - also known affectionately as the "nutritional bypass" - will literally add years to your life.

You will quickly learn that David Rowland is no ordinary nutritionist. He is a trailblazer and trendsetter uninterested in medical buzz terms or fads. Long before Organics were trendy, he was teaching us about the impact of soil depletion. Prior to what has become common knowledge around the link between nutrition and our genes, he was one of the first to address nutritional and biochemical individuality. Well before mainstream began picking up on the importance of detoxification, acknowledging the incidence of gluten sensitivity, appreciating the legitimacy of leaky gut syndrome, the epidemic of inflammation underlying the majority of heart disease, and the infamous Candida connection to common health problems, Rowland has been providing safe and effective holistic solutions for these and hundreds of other conditions. He remains steadfast in upholding and teaching the fundamentals of holistic nutrition and micronutrient supplementation and is able to weed out the junk and provide you with sensible and easy to understand actionable solutions to your health concerns.

Whether your goal is to maintain ideal blood pressure, lower inflammation and free radical burden, learn how to properly measure arterial blockage, manage diabetes and blood sugar, or learn about the best heart healthy fats and oils, by reading this book you can gain new insights into optimizing your heart health. Among other things, this work sheds light on the cholesterol myth and how to unplug your arteries using natural chelation therapy.

The English professor, farmer, novelist, and poet Wendell Berry astutely noted, "People are fed by the food industry, which pays no attention to health, and are treated by the health industry, which pays no attention to food."

David Rowland has made it his calling in life to call attention to this most important issue and help bridge that gap to keep you healthy. **BYPASS the BYPASS:** *Restore Circulation Without Surgery* is incisive and illuminating.

If you've got a heart, and believe your health is an investment and not an expense, turn the page!

Bryce Wylde, B.Sc. Hons., DHMHS
Associate Medical Director at P3Health | CityTV Health Expert |
Medical Advisor DrOZ show | Director My Health Report

Contents

A Lifesaving Breakthrough

In 1983, there were a number of popular dietary supplements in the U.S. that were being promoted for reducing arterial plaque. Although this concept was misnamed "oral chelation", it was based on sound science and had many remarkable successes during its early years. Unfortunately, suppliers starting watering down key ingredients in their products in order to compete with each other on the basis of price. Consumers became disappointed with results, and oral chelation became a short lived fad.

In 1986, I made some scientific improvements to this breakthrough concept, renamed it "arterial cleansing", and introduced it to Canada – where it has been thriving ever since. Countless thousands of people have achieved results not possible by any other method. Fifty-five of them share their experiences with you in this book.

The only way to overcome any health problem is to correct its cause. Drugs and surgery cannot do that. All that modern medicine can do is to alleviate symptoms. Bypass surgery restores circulation temporarily, but does nothing to stop the same or other arteries from plugging up later on. Bypass surgery can do nothing for plugged arteries that are inaccessible to the scalpel, such as behind the heart or in the skull. By correcting the cause of narrowing arteries, however, nutritional arterial cleansing does what the bypass cannot – and much more.

The knowledge in this book can empower you to save or extend your life, or the lives of loved ones. Discover the only sure way of preventing heart attacks and avoiding bypass surgery. Find out how to reduce arterial plaque that has been accumulating for decades. Eliminate angina, shortness of breath, and leg pains while walking. Restore warmth and feeling to hands and feet. Avoid amputation of toes, feet or legs. Arterial cleansing is so successful that it reverses gangrene, something the medical profession cannot do.

From my heart to yours,

David W. Rowland

The Epidemic

Cardiovascular diseases have reached epidemic proportions. They kill more people than all other disease causes combined. Every year, 735,000 Americans have a heart attack, of which 325,000 are fatal. Statistically speaking, *there is about a 44 percent chance your first heart attack will kill you.*

The good news is that these statistics need not apply to you or your loved ones. There is an effective and time tested natural way to correct atherosclerosis, the gradual narrowing of arteries which leads to heart attacks, strokes and gangrene. For over 30 years, many thousands of Canadians have been using this safe and simple method to reduce the deposits in their arteries that have been building up over the years. *This is prevention at its best* – to reverse the cause of the problem before it produces any life-threatening symptoms. Innumerable Canadians have used it to relieve angina and leg pains, to eliminate the need for bypass surgery, and to avoid amputations.

The body has an incredible, innate ability to heal itself, provided we give it the both the raw materials and the conditions it needs to do so. *If you give your body everything it needs, it can heal damaged arteries just as easily as it can heal a cut finger.* This book explains how.

Expect some surprises as you read this book. Cholesterol does <u>not</u> cause heart disease. The first detectable signs of occluding arteries are <u>not</u> fatty streaks. Bypass surgery does <u>not</u> extend lives. Polyunsaturated oils may actually do more harm than good. To paraphrase Will Rogers, *the problem isn't what we don't know; it is what we know that isn't so.*

You are Your Own Healer

Your body is self-repairing. Heart disease has become a rampant killer only because (a) we expose our bodies to hazards at a rate far faster than our natural immune processes can neutralize them, and (b) we do not give our bodies enough of the vital raw materials required to fortify these self-repairing systems. The arterial cleansing program (*aka* "nutritional bypass") answers both of these concerns.

Your body has innate healing wisdom. You can direct the course of your own health without having to trust blindly in anyone else to do it for you. Arterial cleansing gives you the opportunity to improve the quality and perhaps also the length of your life, as it has done and is doing for many thousands of others.

Early Detection

Atheromatous plaque typically builds up on arterial walls gradually, over years and decades. Arteries in vulnerable locations progressively become narrower and narrower – until one day they become so constricted as to precipitate a cardiovascular accident, such as a heart attack or stroke. These events happen when a blood clot or a blob of cholesterol gets stuck in a narrowed opening, or when the artery itself seals shut.

Tissue dies when it is suddenly deprived of its blood supply. If the pacemaker (sinoatrial node) of the heart is affected, then that heart attack is fatal. If other parts of the heart are affected, there is a good chance that the person will survive, given the proper care. Unless the causative atherosclerotic progression is either halted or reversed, however, subsequent heart attacks and/or strokes are likely.

Arteries continue to deteriorate unless and until properly treated with what has been termed, "nutritional arterial cleansing".

Until an artery is about 70% blocked there are usually no symptoms. Unfortunately for many people, the first symptom is death. It is not unusual to hear of someone who has suffered a heart attack within hours or days of having been given a clean bill of health. Stress tests and electrocardiograms can detect only existing and prior heart problems; they cannot predict when a future heart attack may occur.

How Healthy are Your Arteries?

There are a number of early warning signs which indicate deteriorating circulation. Take a moment and check off any that may apply to you:

- ☐ Fingers and/or toes often go cold
- ☐ Arms and/or legs often "go to sleep"
- ☐ Numbness or heaviness in arms or legs
- ☐ Cramps in hand when writing
- ☐ Sharp, diagonal crease in earlobe
- ☐ Tingling sensations in lips or fingers
- ☐ Short walk causes cramping or pains in the legs
- ☐ Memory not as good as it used to be
- ☐ Ankles swell late in the day
- ☐ Breathlessness on slight exertion or on lying down
- ☐ Whitish ring under outer part of cornea in the eye
- ☐ High blood pressure
- ☐ Chest pain after physical exercise or emotional stress

If you have made multiple check marks above – or if you experience even one of these symptoms intensely – your circulatory system is crying out for attention.

Measuring Arterial Blockages

The **coronary angiogram** (arteriogram) has been the most popular coronary diagnostic tool for several decades. The angiogram is a procedure whereby a radioactive dye is injected into the arteries and a film taken to estimate the degree of blockage. If the angiographer reports a 75 percent occlusion of the left main anterior descending artery, surgery is usually recommended. Angiograms can be hazardous. Death rates of up to one percent have been reported. There is a possibility of a heart attack or stroke during the procedure or even months later. There are also risks of torn arteries, infection, and allergic reaction to the dye.

Doppler ultrasound technology: a safe, non-invasive diagnostic method for determining blood flow velocity in coronary, carotid and other arteries. Arterial blockages can actually be seen on a television monitor, the same way that ultrasound is used to show expectant mothers the developing fetus.

Digital pulse analysis (DPA): an indirect method of estimating arterial health. Instead of measuring actual blockages, DPA uses plethysmography to record changes in volume of blood flow and also grades arterial flexibility. The inference is that the less flexible the arteries, the more plaque buildup they have accumulated. DPA has the advantage of being applied in an office setting rather than a hospital. It can be used (a) to indicate the need for arterial cleansing, and (b) to chart one's progress using the Arterial Cleansing Formula.

Symptom amelioration: any symptom that can be quantified is a reliable indicator of progress using the Arterial Cleansing Formula. For example, if initially you could walk only 10 metres before experiencing leg pains and after one month on the ACF you can walk 250 metres without pain, then obviously there has been some reduction in one or more arterial blockages. Similarly, if you used to get angina pains almost daily and now you hardly ever get them, that is tangible evidence of the reduction of at least one coronary artery blockage.

Endoscopic photography: a procedure that involves snaking a tube and optical system into an artery and taking a picture. On the following page are before-and-after photos sent to me by a doctor in Germany. Both photos were taken inside the same coronary artery of the same 68-year old man. The upper photo was taken prior to treatment. The lower was taken after five months on the Arterial Cleansing Formula. (Optimal arterial cleansing in a 68-year old man usually takes about seven months.)

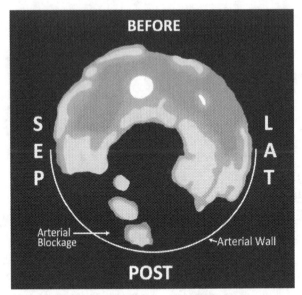

Before: This is an interior photo of a coronary artery in a 68-year old male patient, prior to treatment.

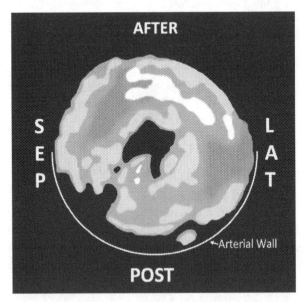

After: This is an interior photo of the same coronary artery in the same 68-year old male patient, after five months of nutritional therapy. This therapy consisted of taking 10 tablets per day of a broad spectrum arterial cleansing formula that includes 16 vitamins, 9 minerals, 2 amino acids and 3 glandular concentrates.

Experience is Proof

In the text boxes that follow are my summaries of 55 of the many reports that have crossed my desk over the years. Most of these people were self-administering their own arterial cleansing programs. Some were assisted by health care practitioners.

Arteries Unblocked
A gentleman who did arterial cleansing for 13 years reported that his arteries were 75% blocked when he started the program and have been totally clear for most of that time.

Active Again
An angiogram showed two blocked arteries with a third being 80% blocked. After seven months of arterial cleansing, this man reported cutting the grass with no stress – and claimed to be living proof that arterial cleansing works. He suggested that he may pass on because of some other disease or accident, but not because of clogged arteries.

Like a New Man
Nine years after the first of five bypass operations, this man's initial symptoms returned. His coronary arteries were found to be from 70 to 90 percent blocked. A sixth bypass was out of the question. After several months of arterial cleansing, he claimed to be feeling like a new man, that he was able to deal with everything.

No More Wheelchair
This lady had been doing arterial cleansing for over 10 years, for blocked arteries affecting mid-thigh of both legs. When she started, she was told that she would never walk again. She now walks where and when she wants, claiming that arterial cleansing keeps her arteries clear and her legs pain free.

Blockages Relieved

A few years after a heart attack, this man was discovered to have a 100% blockage of the circumflex artery and 70% of a main coronary artery. A stent was put in the circumflex artery, but still he was short of breath going up two flights of steps. Nine months after starting arterial cleansing, he claimed to be able to manage two flights of stairs quite well and bicycle almost every day for about 45 minutes without problems.

No More Shakes

This gentleman had three obstructed arteries in his heart, which caused severe weakness and trembling throughout his whole body. With arterial cleansing, he lost his shakiness and claimed to look and feel so much better. Also, his triglycerides came down over 100 points, his blood pressure stabilized, and his cholesterol normalized.

Lives Saved

There are many dietary supplements which have positive benefits for the cardiovascular system, such as: vitamin C, vitamin E, omega-3 oils, L-carnitine, magnesium, coenzyme Q_{10}, garlic, and hawthorne. All of these are beneficial in ameliorating symptoms of cardiovascular diseases. None of these, however, whether taken singly or in combination with any of the others is capable of correcting the cause of arterial blockages. The only dietary supplement known to be able to reduce atherosclerotic buildup is a high potency combination of select vitamins, minerals, amino acids, and glandular concentrates generically known as the "arterial cleansing formula" (ACF). Many people attribute the ACF with saving their lives.

Thank You for All the Years
This man was flat on his back without any income and an 8-year old son. Just two days after starting arterial cleansing, he claimed he could feel it work. Both his feet had been cold, and within a week his right foot warmed up. Then, a week later his left foot warmed up. He attributes arterial cleansing to saving his life and letting him watch his 8-year old grow up to be a 24-year old man.

Saved His Life
Six years after bypass surgery, this gentleman couldn't walk more than 75 yards without nitro-glycerin. Doctors told him that he would live only 6 to 12 months without another bypass, which he refused. Instead, he started on arterial cleansing which in short

order eliminated his leg pain, chest pain, and the need for nitroglycerin. After 8 years of arterial cleansing, this man claims it to be a miracle cure, attributing it with saving his life. He reports that his cardiologist says he is the most outstanding example he knows

Surgeons Baffled by Results
This man had a 5-artery bypass, but three years later his arteries became clogged again. The doctors said, 'Go home and make your will." His circulation was so bad that his toes had turned black and skin was dropping off. He had very little strength, shortness of breath, profound fatigue, and was barely able to walk or do any form of work. Within three months of arterial cleansing, the circulation to his feet improved so much that he stopped wearing socks because his feet were too warm. Six months after he was sent home to die, an angiogram showed that his arteries were as clear as the day the bypass was done. This gentleman attributes arterial cleansing with saving his life.

Saved A Life
This woman attributes arterial cleansing with saving her life. She was diagnosed with atherosclerosis and told that she would die without a bypass operation. Instead, she chose arterial cleansing to treat her condition. She claims it was successful and she is feeling great.

A Life Saved
This lady's husband had a heart attack at age 46. They were horrified when the doctor told them to get his affairs in order. In a health food store, the lady caught sight of my book, *Say 'NO' to Heart Disease*. A tall thin man told her, "If you read that book, I guarantee it will change your life" – which she claims it did. Within three weeks her husband's angina subsided. At the time of writing, her husband was 70 and working three or four days per week. He has his life back.

Diabetes and Gangrene

Anyone with diabetes mellitus is at high risk for cardiovascular accidents. According to the American Heart Association, from 65 to 75 percent of diabetics may die from heart attacks, strokes, or ruptured aneurysms. In addition, diabetics are plagued with impaired peripheral circulation that causes kidney damage (nephropathy), blindness from retinopathy, and amputations of gangrenous toes, feet or even legs. High levels of glucose and insulin in the blood accelerate the development of atherosclerosis, carrying circulatory impairment to extremes.

Diabetic Considerations

It is commonly accepted that high levels of insulin are caustic to the interior wall of arteries, aging them and causing injury that produces plaque. Excess insulin damages arteries and stimulates the synthesis of fats (lipids) in the arterial wall. These fats appear to be formed for purpose of protecting the artery from further injury from the insulin.

When blood sugar is elevated, it produces an increase in the production of the free radicals that cause oxidative damage to arteries and capillaries. This excess production of free radicals happens to everyone after eating a high glycemic meal, usually during only the first half hour while blood sugar is rising. If blood sugar is constantly high, however, there is no relief from the onslaught of free radicals.

Excess glucose in the blood also attaches itself to proteins and fats, altering their structures. This process is referred to as "glycation", which is defined as "the result of co-valent bonding of a protein or lipid molecule with a sugar molecule, such as glucose." Glycation causes proteins in the inner lining of blood vessels to become sticky and to glob together. It also increases the likelihood that bits of plaque may break off and plug up a blood vessel, thus causing a stroke or heart attack.

The Arterial Cleansing Formula includes **chromium** and **magnesium**, both of which minerals help to regulate blood sugar metabolism (glucose tolerance). Some diabetics taking the ACF have been able to reduce their bodies' requirements for insulin injections.

Amputations Avoided

The Arterial Cleansing Formula is the only remedy capable of healing gangrene. Over the last 30 years, many feet and legs have been saved from amputation by taking the ACF.

Leg Saved

Two weeks after vascular surgery was done on this man's left leg, another operation was done near his knee. The surgeon told him that he could do no more; and If the pain got too bad, he should come back to have his leg amputated. After three months of arterial cleansing, his feet were as warm as can be and the sore was gone. He still has his leg.

Both Legs Saved from Amputation
This lady was scheduled for amputation of both legs, due to diabetes. She was told that arterial cleansing may not work quickly enough to avoid surgery. She decided to try arterial cleansing anyway; and after returning to her MD, was told that she no longer needed to have her legs amputated.

Amputation No Longer Required
"I was having considerable difficulty with the circulation in my legs. This was following the advice from the hospital that further bypass operations were impossible. Amputation of my right leg was recommended. A leeway of six months was given ... After seven months of arterial cleansing, I can walk reasonable distances – not fast, but fairly well. I can take in executive length golf courses, etc. This is after terrible discomfort (in the past) within a city block's distance ... I am able to handle most mobile requirements."

Frostbitten Toes Healed
During the coldest part of the winter, this lady froze her right foot. Three toes turned black, with much pain. After one month of arterial cleansing, she claims her foot felt great. No more blackness of toes, and the frozen flesh had been renewed. She claimed to have experienced no more pain or discomfort since.

Pulse Restored
This lady was in the line-up for hip surgery, but was very concerned because the pulse in her legs was not strong. Her doctor was warning of possible complications which could result in amputation. This lady was in her 70s and had weak ankle pulse for several years. After four months of arterial cleansing, she has been told by her doctor that her leg pulse was strong enough to have the hip surgery.

Bypass Surgery

Coronary artery bypass surgery creates a shunt that permits blood to travel from the aorta to a branch of a blocked coronary artery at a point past the obstruction. Since 1968, bypass surgery has been promoted as a life extending procedure. The evidence suggests otherwise.

In 1983, the National Heart, Lung and Blood Institute released its findings of their 10-year Coronary Artery Surgery Study of 780 participants from 15 different hospitals. Results showed that *those who received bypass surgery had no better survival rate than those in similar condition who did not have this surgery*. There was no difference in quality of life between the surgical and non-surgical group. Of those participants selected for surgery, 1.4 percent died during the operation or within 30 days.

A survey at two large military hospitals revealed that 63 percent of patients who underwent coronary bypass surgery before their 36th birthdays either failed to improve, relapsed or died. Of patients aged 45 and over, 45 percent had similarly poor outcomes. [*Medical Abstracts*, Sept/86]

A study of 767 men at several European medical centers showed that *survival rates were no better in many patients who have had coronary bypass surgery than in those who received only drug treatment.* One hundred and nine who had the surgery died within 12 years (compared to 92 in the control group). Thirty-four bypass patients had a total of 44 repeat operations, and five of those 34 died. [*New England Journal of Medicine,* Aug. 11/88]

Bypass surgery performed on the carotid artery is just as questionable. Dr. Henry Barnett, Professor of Neurology at the University of Western Ontario gave a report in Toronto at the July/85 International Congress of Neurologic Surgery. In it he showed, through clinical trial, that carotid bypass surgery (then 20 years old) was worthless. Final analysis of the data showed that patients receiving this surgery had more strokes and fatalities (15%) than similar patients in similar condition who did not receive surgery (4% strokes and fatalities).

Bypass surgery consists of rerouting blood flow around blockages by grafting in a piece of vein taken from elsewhere in the body. The bypass can be performed only on parts of the body that are accessible to the scalpel – such as the front of the heart, the abdomen, or in the neck. ***It is impossible to bypass blood vessels on the back of the heart or in the skull.***

Every surgery has risks. The bypass may have an estimated mortality rate from one to four percent on the operating table, and about 20 percent or more within two years. Sometimes blood clots from the operation migrate and lodge themselves in narrowed arteries elsewhere. Side effects from this operation include strokes, personality changes, decreased IQ, vision loss, and depression.

Any relief that the bypass provides is only temporary. This surgery does nothing to stop blockages from reforming at or near the original site. It does nothing to halt progressive deterioration elsewhere in the arterial tree. One bypass operation often leads to a second or even a third some years down the road. And there is a limit. Sooner or later the body runs out of operable sites.

David Rowland

Other Surgeries

Angioplasty is a less invasive surgical alternative to the bypass. A popular version of this technique involves inserting a balloon catheter into an occluded blood vessel, inflating it, and then rubbing it back and forth to expand the artery and compress the plaque. Another version involves reaming out the blockage with a high speed, very fine drill. A report in the *New England Journal of Medicine* (Sept. 22/88) suggests that in 25 to 40 percent of coronary angioplasty cases, the same vessel becomes blocked again – usually within six months after the procedure.

A **stent** is a stainless steel, self-expanding mesh inserted into a coronary artery. It is typically used to prevent blood vessels from re-closing after bypass surgery or angioplasty.

Surgical methods of treating atherosclerosis attempt either to remove plaque or to bypass plugged arteries, after the damage has been done. *They treat effects but ignore causes.* Unless the atherosclerosis itself is halted, further surgeries are likely to be required.

Bypassing the Bypass
After four hospital stays and numerous tests, this man tried the arterial cleansing. After three months, he told his doctor, a leading cardiologist, about this program. After examination, he was told that his blood pressure was normal and there was no longer any need for coronary bypass surgery. The cardiologist advised him to continue whatever he was doing.

Bypass Avoided for 25 Years
This man had a heart attack almost 30 years before. Although he had numerous angioplasty procedures, he was able to go almost 25 years without a bypass, by taking medication and doing arterial cleansing. His doctors agreed that whatever he was doing has most certainly helped to keep him out of surgery all those years.

Giving Back His Health

Although this man was only 64, he was unable to cope with running a business due to a heart condition which required three separate bypass operations for blockages. He suffered with angina pains that put him into the hospital every few weeks. He could not walk more than a couple of feet without suffering severe shortage of breath; he would have to stop and hold onto something until he felt he could take a few more steps, and stairs were almost an impossibility. He thought he had reached the end of the line when doctors told him he had blockage number four; but this time, because it was located behind his heart, they could do nothing for him. He placed his name with several hospitals for a transplant operation but was turned down as a poor risk. Within a week on arterial cleansing, he started to feel better. Six months later he claimed to feel like a new man. Everyone was amazed at his progress. He could walk around any shopping mall without discomfort, and without any more angina. After returning to the doctor for a thorough checkup, he was told that there were no signs of any blockages and that the fourth blockage behind his heart was also clear. This man was told that his cardiovascular system was in the best shape it had been in, in over 30 years.

Bypass Not Justified

A minister was scheduled for a triple bypass in June. About the middle of April, he started arterial cleansing. Upon the final examination at the end of June, the operation was declared unjustified in view of the patient's recovery.

A Young Man Again

After his second heart attack, this man was told that he would never work again. His cardiovascular surgeon told him that he needed a heart bypass operation but was in such poor shape that he would not survive the operation. He had failing heart valves and coronary arteries that were 90% blocked. His wife had to lift his legs out of bed in the morning. Waking more than a few yards at a time would bring on angina pains. After discovering arterial cleansing, he never looked back. At the time of writing he was in robust health and sometimes walked up to 15 miles a day. His cholesterol count dropped from about 300 to 190, and his blood lipids showed a similar improvement. He claims to have felt like a young man again, enjoying life to the fullest, free from the symptoms of cardiovascular disease which crippled him a few short years before.

Surgery Avoided
This lady had been doing arterial cleansing for several years. Her doctor wanted her to have bypass surgery, but she was able to avoid that. She used to walk on the treadmill for 30 minutes every day but had slowed down a bit. At the time of writing, she was aged 90.

Surgery Not an Option
After suffering from bad circulation in his legs for many years, this man underwent bypass surgery, which he claimed was no laughing matter. After a few years, during a game of tennis, he suddenly felt that fierce pain again. There was no doubt that his arteries had struck back. He could hardly walk a hundred meters. He struggled along for a few more years and had two more bypasses. Each time things went downhill. After the fourth operation, further surgery was not possible. After two weeks of arterial cleansing, however, he started walking more easily. His condition has improved ever since. At the time of writing, he could walk as far as he wanted. Also, cycling was no longer a problem, whereas before he could hardly manage to turn the pedals.

Experimental Surgery Avoided
At the age of 50, this gentleman was told that there was little point in having bypass surgery since it would only increase blood flow to a section of his heart that was already dead. The doctor suggested he consider an experimental procedure that would take a muscle from the back of his shoulder and wrap it around his heart. This muscle would then be jolted by a pacemaker. He declined this

offer. Twenty years later, this man's cardiologist is happy with his heart's performance. He attributes arterial cleansing with having a lot to do with his recovery.

It Works

A lady wrote that the reason her husband's bypass surgery had lasted 22 years is because he had been on arterial cleansing on and off for the last 20 years – and by the way, never changed his diet during all that time.

Chelation Therapy

There is a safe and effective medical technique for removing arterial plaque. It consists of injecting a slow drip solution of magnesium disodium EDTA into a vein over a three hours. It usually takes 30 such treatments (at $100 each) to achieve optimal results. Because EDTA therapy does not correct the cause of the problem, it is wise to repeat this series of injections at regular intervals of every five years or so. Those who take the Arterial Cleansing Formula immediately after EDTA chelation and stay on it consistently should never have the need for a second round of EDTA treatments.

EDTA (ethylene diamine tetraacetic acid) is a synthetic amino acid that binds to minerals in the arterial plaque (calcium, iron, copper, lead, mercury) and removes them from the body. (About 40% of the dry weight of plaques is comprised of calcium.) EDTA is neither altered nor metabolized by the body. Once it binds to a mineral, it is rapidly filtered out by the kidneys into the urine. The EDTA molecule leaves the body intact, bringing minerals with it. Because EDTA is artificial and inert, the body has no need for it and cannot absorb it through the intestinal tract. ***EDTA works <u>only</u> intravenously***.

The word, "chelate", is a chemical term that means to combine with a ring structure, as a claw would grasp an object. Chelation involves the surrounding of mineral or metallic ions by ring structured molecules. The Arterial Cleansing Formula is sometimes referred to as "oral chelation"; however, this term is only a partial description. Although there are a number of nutrients in the ACF which have chelating effects, this nutritional formula works in a number of interrelated ways, perhaps the most significant of which is to act as a "detergent" that dissolves fats in the arterial plaque. The natural chelating factors in the ACF include **L-cysteine**, **DL-methionine**, and **Vitamin C**. There is also **magnesium**, which dissolves calcium deposits – and **vitamin B-1** (thiamine), which facilitates the removal of lead from tissues.

The Arterial Cleansing Formula enables the body to repair underlying damage to the artery walls, by giving the body the raw materials it needs to do its own healing. This is something that EDTA chelation cannot do. Thus, the ACF has the potential to remove more plaque than EDTA therapy can. Some of the plaque has been purposely laid down by the body to patch tears and reinforce weak spots in artery walls. Until those weak areas have been repaired or strengthened nutritionally, the body will <u>not</u> let go of plaque that is required for structural integrity.

Improvement After Chelation

This gentleman received 30 intravenous chelation treatments, and about a month after started nutritional arterial cleansing. Since then he noticed remarkable improvement in his circulation and well-being.

21

Benefits of Arterial Cleansing

Life Extension

Other things being equal, those who achieve excellent health tend to live longer than those who neglect their health. Studies show that bypass surgery does <u>not</u> extend life. There have been no known studies to determine if EDTA chelation therapy extends life. There are, however, many people whose experiences lead them to believe that arterial cleansing has helped them to live longer than they otherwise would have.

Longevity
A lady wrote that she and her husband had been on arterial cleansing for over 20 years and found it very helpful for circulation and for ongoing resistance to colds, flu, etc. Her husband had recently passed at age 84. She believed his longevity to be in part due to arterial cleansing.

Outlived Genealogy
Although this man had heart problems, he outlived all males in his genealogy. He was on arterial cleansing for over 10 years. He believed that it was responsible for keeping his arteries clear and prolonging his life. He also claimed never to get colds, although he used to get many. His father and a younger brother both died 8 to 10 years before they had reached his age.

Angina Relieved

Angina pectoris is severe pain around the heart caused by a relative deficiency of oxygen supply to the heart. It often occurs after increased activity, exercise, or a stressful event. Pain or numbness may radiate to the left shoulder and down the left arm, or it may radiate to the back or jaw. Angina is caused by blockages in one or more coronary arteries and can be relieved by taking the Arterial Cleansing Formula.

"New" Arteries

This 68-year old man suffered an attack of chest pain and was given the usual ECG and stress tests. He was diagnosed with angina and told to come back in two months to discuss bypass surgery. After about two weeks on arterial cleansing, the shortness of breath and the 'pokes' in his chest became less frequent. He was re-examined by a different cardiologist two months later, who could find no evidence of a heart problem. After four months of arterial cleansing, he was able to walk over two miles on a rural road made up of steep hills. The discomfort and warning 'pokes' in the chest had almost entirely disappeared.

No More Angina

This man's angina pectoris, due to hardening of the arteries, became a thing of the past due to arterial cleansing. The pains stopped and his breathing returned to normal. His former lethargy had disappeared, and he claims to have been feeling physically better than he had for many years.

Running Up Stairs

This man had angina and a confirming angiogram that demonstrated extensive coronary stenosis. After being on arterial cleansing for several months, he became pain free and was able to run up and down stairs. His son is a pharmacist who was extremely skeptical that a bunch of vitamins could do anything, but now appears to have done a 180° turn, being convinced that there is something to arterial cleansing that actually works.

Can Walk Farther
After being on arterial cleansing, this woman reports excellent results. A month ago, due to angina, everything was a struggle. To walk one block gave her distress. After three weeks of arterial cleansing, she was walking 20 to 30 blocks as part of her daily exercise program.

Angina Relieved
About a year after being diagnosed with angina, this gentleman had many stress related attacks. The medical doctors assured him that he would need an angiogram and angioplasty; however, he tried arterial cleansing because he felt he had nothing to lose. He claims it kept him free from heart attacks for over 6 months. At the time of writing, he said he was not completely well yet but much better.

Leg Pains Gone

Intermittent claudication is a severe pain in the calf muscles that occurs during walking and subsides with rest. It results from inadequate blood supply, which may be due to atherosclerosis or arterial spasm. Arterial cleansing relieves and eliminates all forms of leg pain that are caused by narrowing arteries.

Surgery Avoided, Pain Gone
This man used to feel pain in the legs after walking only a few hundred meters. After another 10 meters the pain increased so much that he had to stop and wait until the pain ebbed away. He underwent surgery at the groin and everything felt fine again. Years

later, the pain came back, especially in his right leg because a femoral artery was blocked. Again, he underwent surgery. Months later, he felt pain in both legs and also in the neck. Examinations showed that a cervical artery was blocked. Instead of surgery for this, he started arterial cleansing. After one month, the pain in his legs and neck went away. At every six-monthly checkup the doctor keeps telling him that he is all right.

Leg Pains Gone

For over nine months this man was on arterial cleansing, and feeling an enormous improvement. Before starting the treatment, he could not walk 10 meters without feeling an immense pain in the legs. They were also ice cold. At the time of writing, he said that his legs felt good and warm, and that he could easily go out walking. He also remarked that his prostate was functioning better.

Cholesterol Normalized

If you consume a typical western diet, approximately 80 percent of the cholesterol in your blood is made in your own liver. If you are a total vegetarian, then 100 percent of the cholesterol in your blood is made by your liver. This is because cholesterol (a) is found only in animal foods, and (b) is so vital to our wellbeing that the less of it we eat, the more our bodies produce internally. *Elevated and distorted levels of cholesterol have more to do with metabolic imbalances than with dietary intake.*

Many people are able to bring their cholesterol imbalances into line by drinking more water, increasing dietary fibre, eliminating sugar, and getting more exercise. Elevated cholesterol is also one of many possible symptoms of low thyroid function. For those so affected, taking an appropriate level of thyroid hormone restores cholesterol levels to normal.

25

Most people who succumb to heart attacks or strokes, and most of those who have had bypass surgery do __not__ have elevated levels of cholesterol. The usual pattern is for plaque to build up on artery walls without any corresponding change in cholesterol levels in the blood itself. Some people have reported reductions in elevated cholesterol readings as a side benefit of taking the Arterial Cleansing Formula. When this happens, it is most likely because the nutrients in the ACF help to correct whatever metabolic imbalance that was causing the elevated cholesterol.

Cholesterol Lowered
This lady's cholesterol checked out at 237. Her doctor put her on cholesterol medication. She asked her doctor if she could stop taking her cholesterol medicine and instead do arterial cleansing. He said it wouldn't hurt to try, since it is just vitamins. Her cholesterol dropped 58 in just two months on arterial cleansing, without any medication.

Lowering Cholesterol by Clearing Arteries
A natural health practitioner wrote that arterial cleansing is an amazing way to lower cholesterol. It doesn't block cholesterol production but rather corrects the underlying problem (weak or damaged arteries) so the body no longer needs to make cholesterol to fix the damage. She used it successfully with her patients, claiming that their arteries are no longer occluded, as verified by MRI - and adding that the medical doctors are always amazed.

Cholesterol and Blood Pressure Down
A colon hydrotherapist uses arterial cleansing in conjunction with her treatments. To date, all of her clients (except one), in 11 years of practice, no longer have to take their high cholesterol or high blood pressure medication."

Healthy Cholesterol
This man claims that arterial cleansing has kept his cholesterol LDL:HDL a healthy ratio. He no longer takes prescribed statins, which he claims actually have more negative side effects than the 'potential' result of lowering cholesterol. Arterial cleansing has been part of his daily regime for over 5 years.

Blood Pressure Normalized

Most cases of high blood pressure (hypertension) are caused or aggravated by hidden food allergies. Almost any food or beverage can cause this response, depending on each person's unique sensitivities. The most frequent offenders in this regard, however, are caffeine and the nightshade family (tomatoes, potatoes, peppers, paprika, eggplant, cayenne, and tobacco). Blood pressure usually returns to normal within four days of eliminating 100 percent of the causative allergens.

Sometimes hypertension is also caused by narrowing arteries that are losing flexibility. The heart has to pump harder in order to assure that the blood flows everywhere it can, causing blood pressure to increase. In such cases, arterial cleansing tends to restore blood pressure to normal.

Blood Pressure Lowered
This 59-year old man been taking blood pressure drugs for about two years. After three weeks of arterial cleansing, his blood pressure was down considerably. In no time he was off blood pressure medication. He was very happy with the results, claiming to feel 100% better.

Heart Function

The cardiac muscles of the heart receive their blood supply through two or more branched coronary arteries. Accumulating blockages in any of these small arteries eventually cause angina and heart attacks. Reducing such blockages before any adverse symptoms are experienced may be considered prevention rather than therapy. Such prevention does <u>not</u> improve the function of the heart but rather maintains its *status quo* by keeping it from deteriorating.

Arterial cleansing is only of indirect benefit to structural abnormalities within the heart itself. Reducing blockages throughout the arterial tree eases the load on the heart: this muscular organ does not have to work quite so hard if it is no longer pushing against obstructions. There have been a few cases in which it appears that the chelating ingredients in the ACF may have reduced calcification on heart valves. Heart murmurs, however, do <u>not</u> respond to arterial cleansing.

and going on arterial cleansing. The ejection fraction of her left ventricle increased to 49 percent, which improvement she attributes to arterial cleansing.

General Health

Optimal arterial cleansing enables the body to reduce and eliminate arterial plaque wherever it may occur. Doing so enables the circulatory system to become more efficient, improving the blood's ability to bring oxygen and nutrients to bodily cells everywhere. The result is improved overall health.

Kept in Good Health for 30 Years
This couple was on arterial cleansing for almost 30 years and credit their health successes to this program. They both depend on it, claiming that It has kept them in good health and nothing else works as well.

Walking and Climbing Stairs Again
A 75-year old man suffered from arteriosclerosis in the neck and legs. After an emergency operation, things went from bad to worse. He had an embolism and lost the sight in his left eye. Walking was out of the question and climbing stairs was pure torture. After four months of arterial cleansing, he felt much better. Every day he walks for a half hour, and climbing stairs is no longer a problem. He also cycles every day 5 to 10 km on an exercise bicycle.

Kept Me Going
This person wrote that arterial cleansing has kept her going for about 20 years.

20 Years Younger
Another wrote that he does arterial cleansing, is 70 years old and can keep up with any 50-year old.

Feel 100%
This man claims that arterial cleansing has cleaned out his system, like flushing a radiator. Six months after his heart attack, doctors couldn't understand why it happened because his arteries were so clear. He claims to have the blood pressure of an 18-year old, with a heart rate that is fantastic, and feeling 100 percent all round.

84 Years Young
This man had been doing arterial cleansing for 11 years. The last test done on his arteries showed them to be clear of plaque. At the time of writing, he was aged 84, conducting two orchestras, playing in the symphony, and teaching privately.

Younger, Healthier, Happier
Three stents were inserted into this man's coronary arteries. Since being on arterial cleansing, there was no further deterioration – only improvement. Circulation to his left index finger was fully restored, and his swollen ankles became a thing of the past. These were his observations of the results: improved blood sugar levels, stamina, general sense of well-being, and skin tone – got him back into the gym, doing 45 minutes at a time on the treadmill – helped reduce his medications – stopped his sugar cravings – prevented him from having to have another stent or further surgical intervention – no more being rushed to hospital by ambulance – increased libido – and being far happier with far less sense of being old and washed up.

In Very Good Health
This lady was on arterial cleansing for several years – which she claimed kept her in very good health, with friends and family marveling at the energy she had that kept her active in the family, the church and the community. She attributed this to arterial

cleansing. At the time of writing, she was 73 years of age, a mother of four. and grandmother of six.

Prescription Drugs Avoided
Prior to arterial cleansing, this lady's husband was having heart, blood pressure, and cholesterol issues. On arterial cleansing he was able to avoid using any prescription drugs.

Other Benefits

The entire body benefits from improved circulation. Sometimes arterial cleansing produces unexpected rewards – such as higher energy levels, improved vision, better prostate function, or increased libido.

Pounding Sensations Gone
This lady went on arterial cleansing to get relief from the debilitating conditions of fatigue plus a pounding sensation in her head. She was happy to say that after following the program for 10 days, the pounding sensation in her head stopped and never returned.

Vision Improved
This 89-year old lady had great results with the arterial cleansing that she had been doing for over two years. Her arteriosclerosis improved, and when she went for a recent eye test, her results were so good that the doctor could not believe he was looking at the eyes of an 89-year old.

Sexual Abilities Renewed
This 46-year old man was on arterial cleansing for six months at the time, and very pleased with the results. His main problem was a genetic predisposition to very high cholesterol levels. He was also having problems with erectile dysfunction. His hormone levels

had been checked and testosterone found to be normal. Arterial cleansing, controlling his eating habits, exercising regularly, and drinking lots of spring water apparently renewed his sexual abilities. He felt that the problem was resolved by cleansing the blood vessels that were blocked.

The Cholesterol Myth

If you believe that normal cholesterol levels protect you from getting a heart attack, you may be dead wrong – literally. No matter how carefully you follow a low-cholesterol diet, no matter how much butter or how many eggs you avoid, your chances of dying prematurely from a heart attack are about the same as if you had <u>not</u> restricted your cholesterol intake.

The cholesterol-as-cause notion is pseudoscientific nonsense. Cholesterol is a major component of the plaque that occludes arteries; however, cholesterol is a later constituent that is laid down in the plaque, not the first. *Cholesterol is a slippery, waxy substance that cannot possibly adhere to a smooth, healthy arterial lining.* (Similarly, fats cannot stick to a healthy arterial lining.)

There is just as much cholesterol circulating in our veins as in our arteries, but plaque is found only in arteries and never in veins. If cholesterol were the cause of circulatory impairment, then surely it would damage veins as much as arteries. But clearly it does <u>not</u>.

Epidemiological evidence refutes the cholesterol myth. The first heart attack documented in medical records occurred in 1910. For a century or more prior to that time, the typical western diet, especially in rural areas, consisted of relatively large quantities of eggs, butter, lard, bacon, sausage, pork – and no one died from heart disease.

Cholesterol is a vital bodily substance. It is in every cell in the body. Cholesterol helps to conduct nerve impulses; 17 percent of brain tissue is cholesterol. It is a constituent of bile. Cholesterol is a component of cellular membranes and a number of hormones, including the sex hormones. It also helps to manufacture vitamin D under the skin, in response to sunlight. *Cholesterol is so important that the less of it we eat, the more our bodies produce.* As mentioned earlier, for those of us on omnivorous diets, the body produces about 80 percent of the cholesterol it needs internally, with only 20% coming from food consumed. For those of us who are total vegetarians (vegans), 100 percent of bodily cholesterol is produced by the body itself.

There is no direct correlation between serum cholesterol levels and the incidence of coronary artery disease. *Various reports suggest that anywhere from 50 to 80 percent of those who have heart attacks or bypass surgery do not have elevated cholesterol levels.* Over the years, I have interviewed a number of doctors and nurses on cardiac teams, all of whom concur that most heart attacks occur in people whose cholesterol levels are within normal range.

In 1953, Ancel Keys published a report showing a supposed correlation between the consumption of fats/cholesterol and the incidence of heart disease in six countries. Mr. Keys committed selection bias, however, because he had data from 22 countries but chose only those six which supported his preconceived notion. One of the countries he excluded was France, which has both a high consumption of fat and a low incidence of heart disease. Had Keys plotted all 22 sets of data, there would have been no correlation whatsoever, simply random points on a graph. Keys was not the only researcher to manipulate or misinterpret statistics. *All of the studies allegedly implicating cholesterol as the cause for heart disease are based on either flawed research or results which are statistically insignificant.* [*The Cholesterol Myths*, Uffe Ravnskov, MD, PhD]

The misplaced focus on dietary cholesterol has diverted attention away from an important discovery: *both cholesterol and triglyceride levels tend to rise more in response to dietary sugars, caffeine and alcohol than they do in response to dietary fats or*

cholesterol. Often serum cholesterol can be brought back to normal by the complete elimination of concentrated sweets (e.g., sugar, candy, pastries, cookies, soda pop, etc.), caffeine (e.g., coffee, tea colas) and alcoholic beverages.

A Scientific Explanation

Science is the intellectual process using all available mental and physical resources to better understand, explain, and predict normal as well as unusual natural phenomena. The scientific approach to understanding anything involves observation, measurement of that which can be quantified, and the accumulation of data.

Empirical science is based on, concerned with, or verifiable by observation or experience rather than theory or pure logic. The law of gravity was discovered and is completely verifiable by observation and experience, as is the fact that the earth revolves around the sun, and also the fact that citrus juices cure scurvy.

Epidemiology is that branch of science concerned with the incidence and distribution of health related states and events in populations. Epidemiology tells us that *atherosclerosis has reached epidemic proportions and kills more people than all other disease causes combined*.

From the above perspectives, the Arterial Cleansing Formula (ACF) is on a solid scientific footing. Many, many thousands of people have been using this formula over a 30-year time period to remove arterial blockages, as evidenced by amelioration of their symptoms (e.g., no more angina, bypass surgery avoided, intermittent claudication gone, no more tingling sensations, warmer hands/feet, gangrene reversed) as well as by confirming ultrasound tests of coronary and carotid arteries. *This is both empirical and epidemiological evidence of outstanding significance*.

Repeatability and predictability are the reasons science exists. When event A happens, we want to know what the outcome will be. The ACF meets all scientific standards of predictability. We know what happens when people take it. *The ACF is to atherosclerosis what oranges are to scurvy.*

Experiential Proof

Experience is the ultimate proof. We know for a fact that the Arterial Cleansing Formula works because of its incredible history of successes. Because of biochemical individuality, responses to this formula vary from person to person. Those who are in reasonably good health may experience only subtle benefits, while others can overcome significant health conditions, thereby extending their lives and improving their quality of life. There have been only about 25 individuals over the last 30 years that have reported no perceptible benefits from taking the ACF. The only way to know if the ACF will work for you is to try it. The answer to the question, "What proof do you have that the ACF works?" is, "Take it and you will be the proof."

Humanity has been blessed with inquiring minds. Sometimes knowing that something works is not enough. We want to know why or how, and such questioning leads us into the realm of theory. ("Theory" is a fancy word for "supposition".)

Theories come and go. At various times in history scientists believed that the world was flat, that the sun revolved around the earth, that bloodletting was a cure-all for whatever ails you, and that cholesterol causes heart disease. All four of these theories are false. *The truth of an idea has nothing to do with its popularity. Sometimes the majority can be wrong.*

Once a notion becomes entrenched in one's thinking, it can be difficult to see other possibilities. The tendency is to see only what you wish. Scientists refused to look through the lens of Galileo's "foolish" telescope because they were absolutely certain that the sun revolved around the earth. French doctors in the time of Jacques Cartier refused to believe that his men had been cured from scurvy by consuming pine needle tea. They said, "No. That can't work. That's witchcraft."

First Evidence of Damage

The first visual evidence we have of developing atherosclerosis is *what mistakenly appear to be* fatty streaks in the inner lining of arteries. Closer examination reveals that these streaks are <u>not</u> fats but rather dead macrophages (immune cells). These macrophages have become trapped in rough scar tissue caused by the healing of tiny cuts or tears in the arterial lining. Thus, ***the true cause of atherosclerosis is whatever damages the arterial wall.*** The most likely suspects are free radicals, homocysteine, and diabetes.

Oxidized Cholesterol

A number of scientists who became disenchanted with the cholesterol theory decided to modify it somewhat. They observed that not all cholesterol in arterial deposits is the same; some of it has become oxidized. They speculated that it must be the oxidized cholesterol that causes the damage; and from this assumption followed a number of dietary precautions, such as cooking eggs over low heat so as not to damage their cholesterol content.

The oxidized cholesterol theory has two flaws: (1) oxidized cholesterol is one of the last ingredients laid down in the arterial plaque, not the first, and (2) it is more likely that this cholesterol became oxidized after it accumulated in the plaque. An outer layer of cholesterol may have sacrificed itself in order to protect deeper layers and the artery itself from the damaging effects of oxygen free radicals. From this perspective, cholesterol could be considered an antioxidant of last resort.

Inflammation

<u>Inflammation</u> is a nonspecific immune response that occurs in reaction to any type of bodily injury. C-reactive protein (CRP) is a protein found in the blood, the levels of which rise in response to inflammation and are associated with atherosclerosis, diabetes, autoimmune disorders and sports injuries. In other words, atherosclerosis raises CRP levels, but not all elevated CRP levels are triggered by atherosclerosis.

Arterial inflammation usually increases CRP levels before any significant blockages show up on ultra sound tests. This does not mean that inflammation causes atherosclerosis, however. Jumping to this kind of erroneous conclusion is known in logic as the *post hoc proper hoc* fallacy – meaning that just because one event precedes another does not prove that the former caused the latter. In scientific terms, this is the error of assuming that correlation is cause.

Inflammation is an effect, <u>not</u> a cause. Inflammation does not cause atherosclerosis any more than inflammation causes arthritis or sports injuries. In all cases, inflammation is a response to damage of some kind. We need to find out what is causing the damage. With respect to atherosclerosis, the most likely causative agents are free radicals, homocysteine and elevated blood glucose (as in diabetes).

Hypoascorbemia

Humans, apes, guinea pigs, and fruit-eating bats all suffer from a genetic mutation whereby they do <u>not</u> produce ascorbate (vitamin C) in their livers the way other mammals do. What we call vitamin C is really a liver metabolite that participates in many biochemical pathways in the body.

Dr. Irwin Stone postulated that scurvy was not a dietary disturbance, but a potentially fatal flaw in human genetics that has been misunderstood by nutritionists. He proposed the name, "hypoascorbemia", for the effects of this genetic defect. He proposed that ascorbate is not a vitamin required only in trace amounts, but is required by humans in relatively large daily quantities.

Hypoascorbemia (insufficent vitamin C) is the reason why sailors used to develop scurvy on long voyages on which they were deprived of fresh fruits and vegetables. Hypoascorbemia is the reason why supplementary vitamin C is beneficial to so many health conditions. It is also the reason why research monkeys die if they are not given 70 times the equivalent amount of vitamin C recommended for humans [*Linus Pauling, PhD, at a lecture given in Toronto, circa 1985*].

Here is a remarkable fact: **animals which produce ascorbate in their livers are immune to atherosclerosis.** If you wish to induce atherosclerosis in animals for research purposes, you have to use monkeys or guinea pigs. Somehow, the ability to produce vitamin C internally prevents an animal's arteries from plugging up. This is probably due to at least three biochemical mechanisms: (1) vitamin C is required for the production of lipoprotein lipase (LPL), an arterial cleansing enzyme, (2) vitamin C is required for the production of Co-enzyme Q_{10}, an antioxidant that protects arteries from damaging oxygen free radicals, and (3) vitamin C is itself a powerful antioxidant.

If the human liver were capable of producing vitamin C in the same way that other animals' livers do, it would probably produce a range of from 2,000 mg to 10,000 mg per day, when converted for equivalent body weight, the higher amounts being required during times of stress. The implication is that by taking suitably high amounts of vitamin C throughout our entire lives, we may be able to prevent atherosclerosis. It is unlikely, however, that vitamin C supplementation alone would be capable of removing arterial plaque that has been accumulating over years.

Lipoprotein Lipase

Cholesterol, triglycerides and phospholipids are lipoproteins, the molecules of which consist of fats chemically linked to proteins. Lipoproteins are classified as very low-density (VLDL), low-density (LDL), intermediate density (IDL), and high density (HDL). It is thought that individuals with high blood levels of HDL are less predisposed to coronary heart disease than those with high blood levels of VLDL or LDL. This is because the lower density lipoproteins are puffier and tend to more easily block openings in tiny capillaries or in arteries that have become narrowed by pre-existing plaque. The body's natural way of reducing excess lipoproteins is to make lipoprotein lipase (LPL).

Lipoprotein lipase (LPL) is a water soluble, fat splitting enzyme (i.e., an emulsifier) that hydrolyzes triglycerides in lipoproteins, such as those found in very low density lipoproteins (VLDL) in the blood, into free fatty acids and one monoacylglycerol molecule. LPL is also involved in promoting the cellular uptake of chylomicron remnants, cholesterol-rich lipoproteins, and free fatty acids. LPL is attached to the surface of some cells that line the capillaries and arteries, and is also distributed in adipose, heart and skeletal muscle tissue, as well as in lactating mammary glands.

Lipoprotein lipase works like a detergent to emulsify excess cholesterol and triglycerides, breaking them down and enabling them to be carried safely away through the liver and bile. There is a catch, however. The body requires an abundant supply of vitamin C in order to be able to produce enough LPL to do its job. This ascorbate-LPL dependence may be one of the mechanisms by which most animals are protected from atherosclerosis and we humans are not. Without a sufficiently high intake of **vitamin C**, the human body cannot produce enough LPL to prevent excess fats and cholesterol from accumulating in arterial plaque.

Lipoprotein(a)

Lipoprotein(a) is structurally similar to low density lipoproteins (LDL) and is often considered to be a marker for atherosclerotic diseases. If there is a significant lipoprotein(a) reading in your blood work, you are theoretically considered to be at higher risk of developing atherosclerosis than if your other lipoprotein fractions are out of balance. But there is a missing link in this chain of reasoning. Lipoprotein(a) may well indicate a genetic predisposition for elevated or distorted cholesterol readings. However, there is no conclusive scientific evidence that cholesterol or other lipoproteins actually cause atherosclerosis, plus a number of logical reasons why they cannot. [*See "The Cholesterol Myth" above.*]

Co-Enzyme Q_{10}

Co-enzyme Q_{10} (ubiquinone, ubiquinol) is a vitamin-like substance that is present in all bodily cells and generates energy in the form of adenosine triphosphate (ATP). CoQ_{10} is present in large amounts in those organs with the highest energy requirements, namely the heart, liver and kidneys. CoQ_{10} also functions as an antioxidant to protect cells against the damaging effects of oxygen free radicals. These combined actions of CoQ_{10} help both to strengthen the heart muscle and to prevent damage to arterial walls.

Internal production of CoQ_{10} is ascorbate dependant, which may be another of the reasons why most animal's bodies are protected against atherosclerosis, whereas those with hypoascorbemia are not. If the body has a sufficiently high intake of **vitamin C** and **B-vitamins**, it may be capable of producing all of the CoQ_{10} it needs – without resorting to dietary CoQ_{10}. Large amounts of vitamin C can also supplement and even replace the antioxidant activity of CoQ_{10}. Cholesterol lowering drugs interfere with and deplete the body's production of CoQ_{10}, however, so anyone taking these pharmaceuticals is well advised also to take supplementary CoQ_{10}.

Free Radicals

A <u>free radical</u> is an unstable, highly reactive molecular fragment that contains an odd number of electrons and an open bond or half bond. If two radicals meet, both are eliminated. If a radical reacts with a nonradical, another free radical is produced. This type of event becomes a chain reaction and contributes to the development of ischemic injury, such as myocardial infarction (heart attack). Cascading free radical reactions appear to be the most significant cause of arterial damage.

Homocysteine

Homocysteine is a toxic amino acid that irritates and damages artery walls. Homocysteine is an intermediate by-product resulting from the incomplete breakdown (catabolism) of methionine, an amino acid that is abundant in our diet.

A high level of homocysteine in the blood (hyperhomocysteinemia) is associated with an increased risk of developing coronary artery disease, and may account for 60 percent of peripheral vascular diseases (i.e., those affecting the extremities). Men with hyperhomocysteinemia may have three times more heart attacks than those with low levels of homocysteine.

The ideal level of homocysteine in the blood is zero, and it is very easy to achieve this level. All that is necessary is to take sufficient levels of **vitamin B_6**, **vitamin B_{12}**, and **folic acid** – all of which vitamins are generously supplied in the ACF (Arterial Cleansing Formula).

Blood Sugar

All of the various sugars we consume are first broken down in the digestive tract into the simple sugars glucose (dextrose) and fructose (levulose), then immediately absorbed through the intestinal wall directly into the bloodstream. The liver converts fructose into glucose, so ultimately every kind of sugar ends up as glucose (blood sugar). If we consume too much sugar, our blood becomes flooded with excess levels of glucose. If our pancreas, liver and adrenal glands are in fine working order, then this spike in blood sugar is only temporary. If our endocrine system is out of balance and we push our sugar consumption, then we may develop hypoglycemia or diabetes. (Some forms of diabetes are caused or aggravated by genetic weakness.)

Hypoglycemia is characterized by compulsive sugar consumption which triggers multiple highs and lows in blood sugar throughout the day. In diabetes, blood sugar is constantly too high. Unfortunately, ***high glucose levels accelerate free radical damage*** – the degree of which damage is most probably in direct proportion to how high the glucose level and for how much of the day. In the development of arterial damage (a) diabetes is an accelerating factor, (b) hypoglycemia is probably an aggravating factor, and (c) in otherwise healthy people, high sugar meals may cause some degree of arterial stress. Our bodies can get all of the glucose we need for optimal functioning from the gradual breakdown of complex carbohydrates (e.g., whole grains, starchy vegetables), thus avoiding spikes in blood sugar.

Blood Fats

The body has a very clever way of assuring that fats in the bloodstream stay within an acceptable range. The fats that we consume are broken down by the action of bile and **lipase** enzymes into simpler fatty acids that are absorbed into the lymphatic system rather than into the blood. To absorb fats directly into the bloodstream would be fatal. Instead, fats circulate throughout the lymphatics and are transferred into the blood on an 'as needed' basis. Thus, the <u>quantity</u> of fats in the blood is strictly regulated and is of no consequence to atherosclerosis. The <u>quality</u> of fats, however, significantly affects arterial health. Unstable polyunsaturated oils, rancid fats and *trans* fats circulating in our lymphatic system find their way into cellular membranes, thus increasing their vulnerability to free radical damage.

Composition of Arterial Plaque

<u>Atheroma</u> is an accumulation and swelling in artery walls made up of macrophage cells, debris, lipids (cholesterol and fatty acids), calcium and a variable amount of fibrous connective tissue. These accumulations are commonly referred to as atheromatous plaques. It is an unhealthy condition, but is found in most humans. ***Veins do <u>not</u> develop atheromata***, unless surgically moved to function as an artery, as in bypass surgery.

The <u>atheromatous swelling</u> is always between the endothelium lining and the smooth muscle wall central region (media) of the arterial tube. While the early stages (based on appearance) have traditionally been termed fatty streaks by pathologists; they are <u>not</u> composed of fat cells, but instead are accumulations of white blood cells, especially macrophages. After accumulating large amounts of cytoplasmic membranes (with associated high cholesterol content), these dead macrophages are called, "foam cells". When foam cells die, their contents are released, which attracts more macrophages and creates an extracellular lipid core near the center to inner surface of each atherosclerotic plaque. The outer, older portions of the plaque become calcified.

Visually, the thickening of the walls of the arteries appears as an accumulation of soft, flaky, yellowish material with deposits of swollen macrophages as its bottom layer and a somewhat firmer coating on top. Interspersed in this accumulation can be seen fibrous tissue, calcium, cholesterol crystals, and fatty material. Some plaques are unstable and can rupture. Because of its spontaneous abnormal growth and swelling, plaque loosely fits the definition of a benign tumour.

Macrophages are the major scavenger immune cells in the blood, which clear it of diseased cells, cellular debris and pathogenic organisms. The question is why do macrophages make up such a large part of the atherosclerotic plaque? Why also are these white blood cells the first constituent of plaque to adhere to the artery wall? The clearest answer to both questions is that the macrophages are needed to dispose of arterial cells that have become damaged. Macrophages absorb damaged proteins and LDL cholesterol, then swell up to become foam cells that stick to the injured artery wall. The **vitamin A** and **thymus** concentrate in the ACF enable the thymus gland to increase production of macrophages, thus facilitating the cleanup of damaged arterial cells.

What is this fibrous connective tissue that is also a significant component of arterial plaque? Most probably it is the result of blood platelets doing their job. When a blood vessel is injured, platelets adhere to each other and the edges of the injury to form a plug that covers the area. This leads to enhancement of the coagulation mechanism and deposition of fibrin. The plug that is formed acts like a scab which retracts to stop the loss of blood The actions of platelets, although quite beneficial in initiating the reaction to injury, may actually be harmful in conditions such as coronary occlusion. In that case, platelet function may delay restoration of the blood supply and help to cause re-occlusion of the vessel. Healthy platelets are critical to the healing of the artery wall; but unhealthy platelets tend to stick to each other excessively, thus adding unnecessary bulk to the arterial plaque. **Vitamin E** keeps platelets healthy and prevents them from unduly sticking together.

Fibrin is a whitish, filamentous protein that is the basis for blood clotting. This fibrin is deposited as fine interlacing filaments, containing entangled red and white blood cells and platelets, the whole forming a coagulum or clot. Fibrinogen is the protein in blood plasma that is converted into fibrin by the action of thrombin and in the presence of calcium ions. In other words, fibrin acts like a scab to prevent a cut or tear from bleeding out or hemorrhaging – and also traps calcium ions before they can form lumps of calcium that would plug arteries and capillaries. This rough scab-like structure on the artery wall becomes a matrix in which are trapped minerals, heavy metals, macrophages, cellular debris, fats, and cholesterol from the bloodstream – *substances that could not possibly adhere to the smooth lining of a healthy artery.*

Minerals and fats attract each other, because of opposing electromagnetic charges. Minerals from the bloodstream become trapped in arterial scar tissue and attract fats electromagnetically. These fats become an integral part of the accumulating plaque, and in turn attract more minerals, especially calcium – and so on, repeating the cycle and ever increasing the size of the plaque.

Cellular Integrity

Atherosclerosis occurs only in arteries, never in veins. This is because of the structural differences between artery cells and vein cells.

Every cell in our bodies is enclosed in a membrane that separates the interior of cells from their outside environment. This cellular membrane selectively controls which molecules may enter and exit the cell. The basic function of the cellular membrane is to protect the cell from its surroundings.

Most cellular membranes consist of about 50% lipids (fats), depending on the type of cell. These lipids are in two layers which behave as fluids in which individual molecules (both lipids and proteins) are free to rotate and move. Such fluidity of membranes is greatly affected by lipid composition. Lipids containing unsaturated fatty acids increase membrane fluidity because the presence of loose double carbon bonds introduces kinks in the fatty acid chains, making them more difficult to pack together. Cholesterol in membranes also increases fluidity. What all this means is that *the more unsaturated fatty acids and cholesterol a cellular membrane contains, the more fluid or flexible it is.*

Because monounsatured fatty acids (i.e., omega-9) have only one double carbon bond in their structure, they are more stable and less fluid than unsaturated fatty acids. Thus, *omega-9 fatty acids contribute stability to cellular membranes.* Oleic acid is the primary omega-9 fatty acid in our cellular membranes and is provided in large amounts by olive oil, almond oil, macadamia oil, avocado oil and cashew oil.

Arteries are the high pressure tubes of the circulatory system. They contain an extra muscular layer that the veins do not. These arterial muscles are constantly flexing, pushing blood along. In order to maintain this flexibility, artery cells have to be more fluid than most other cells in the body – meaning that they necessarily have to contain a relatively high percentage of unsaturated fats – and therein lies their vulnerability. *Unsaturated fats are unstable and highly susceptible to free radical damage* because of the large number of weak double carbon bonds in their molecular structure.

In order to maintain necessary flexibility, artery cells contain a high proportion of unstable unsaturated fats and a low percentage of the stable, protective monounsaturates. The body does its best to maintain a favourable ratio of unsaturates to monounsaturates in arterial cells; however, its ability to do so is limited by diet. If we do not consume enough monounsaturates, then the body has no choice but to fill cellular membranes with even more unsaturates than is healthy or desirable, thus making the arteries structurally weaker and more vulnerable to free radical damage than they would otherwise be. ***The more polyunsaturated oils we consume, the weaker our arteries become, unless we also increase our intake of the protective monounsaturates accordingly.***

It is ironic that the highly promoted polyunsaturated oils (e.g., safflower, sunflower, corn, soy, walnut, flax, pumpkin) may actually contribute to the development of atherosclerosis if consumed to excess. Consistent with this theory is epidemiological evidence which shows that in Mediterranean countries where olive oil (79% monounsaturates) is a staple, the incidence of heart disease is significantly lower than it is elsewhere.

Collateral Circulation

If a blood clot suddenly plugs up a narrowed coronary artery, this immediate deprivation of blood usually causes an instant heart attack. If the blood supply to the heart's internal pacemaker is suddenly cut off, then that heart attack is fatal. If other areas of the heart are suddenly deprived of blood, and provided the damage is not too extensive, the result is usually a non-fatal heart attack.

If a coronary artery narrows gradually and provided there is enough **vitamin E** present, the body is often able to develop collateral circulation: it gradually extends other arteries and capillaries into the area that is slowly being deprived of its usual blood supply. This phenomenon was discovered during autopsies and cardiac surgeries which revealed previously unknown arterial blockages for which the body had created its own bypasses.

The body has its own wisdom of timing in creating collateral circulation. Blood vessels are extended into the vulnerable area before they are required. Then, when the coronary artery seals shut, it is a non event. The heart remains fully functional.

Recently, a client reported to me that two of his coronary arteries were discovered to be 100 percent blocked, yet he had no symptoms. He passed two stress tests with flying colors, hardly breaking a sweat and without any shortness of breath. His cardiologist told him everything was great, that collateral circulation had kept his heart healthy.

Arterial Spasms

Apart from accumulating plaque, arteries can fail in an entirely different way. Spasms in otherwise healthy coronary arteries can temporarily restrict blood supply to the heart, causing angina, a heart attack, and/or death. In death, the artery relaxes so that an autopsy will be unable to find any apparent cause for the heart attack. **Magnesium** prevents arterial spasms.

A Plausible Theory

From the above observations we can piece together a theory that (a) is more plausible than any others advanced to date, and (b) is consistent with our successful experience with arterial cleansing. There are three parts to this theory: (1) atherosclerosis is caused by agents that damage artery walls, (2) the body does what it can to control the damage, the unfortunate consequence of which is the accumulation of plaque that gradually occludes arteries, and (3) certain high potency nutrients can enable the body both to prevent arterial occlusion and also to reverse that which has already taken place.

Key elements in this theory:

- Free radicals and homocysteine create tiny tears in the inner lining of artery walls.
- Excess blood sugar accelerates this arterial damage.
- The body patches arterial tears with fibrin (a clotting protein) and scarring.

- Dead macrophages (immune cells) become trapped in the patches and scar tissue.
- These macrophages swell up to become foam cells.
- Through time, more and more substances become attracted to and trapped in the arterial patches – including collagen, fats, minerals (especially calcium), foreign proteins, heavy metals, phospholipids, mucopolysaccharides, muscle tissue, cellular debris, triglycerides, and cholesterol.
- The parts of the arterial tree most vulnerable to the accumulation of plaque are the coronary arteries, the carotid arteries, and the femoral arteries.
- Plaque that is allowed to proliferate out of control will eventually cause a heart attack, a stroke, or gangrene.
- **Antioxidants** protect the arteries from the damaging effects of oxygen free radicals. (An antioxidant is a molecule that can absorb a renegade electron without becoming a free radical itself.) Dietary antioxidants include **vitamin C**, **vitamin E**, and **selenium**.
- **Vitamin C** and the **B-vitamins** encourage the body to make coenzyme Q_{10}, an internally generated antioxidant.
- **Selenium**, **zinc** and **manganese** facilitate the body's production of free radical scavengers.
- **Vitamins B_6, B_{12}** and **folic acid** eliminate the homocysteine hazard.
- **Vitamin C** in large amounts encourages the arteries to produce LPL, an enzyme that emulsifies and disposes of fats that have accumulated in artery walls.
- Certain high potency nutrients act as chelating agents to remove minerals and heavy metals from arterial plaque – including **vitamin C**, **L-cysteine**, **DL-methionine**, and **thiamine** (vitamin B-1).
- **Magnesium** dissolves calcium deposits in arterial plaque.
- **Magnesium** also prevents arterial spasms, some of which can be fatal.

- Large amounts of **vitamin E** encourage the body to develop collateral circulation, in effect creating self-generated bypasses.

- **Choline** emulsifies fats, keeping them from sticking together and thereby improving the flow characteristics of the blood.

- **Vitamin E** prevents blood platelets from sticking together, thus reducing their tendency to contribute to excessive coagulation in arterial patches.

- **Monounsaturated oils** (e.g., olive, avocado, almond) have a protective effect on arterial cell membranes.

Free Radicals

Free radicals are the most likely causative agents for atherosclerosis. These are highly unstable molecular fragments with unpaired electrons in their outer orbits, causing them to react instantly with substances in their vicinity, damaging cells and creating abnormal cells. Oxygen free radicals are especially dangerous because they react readily with other molecules. This is why we need antioxidants, agents that protect cells from the damaging effects of peroxides and superoxide (highly reactive forms of oxygen).

The body produces enzymes which act as free radical "scavengers", whose role is to neutralize as many free radicals as possible before they can cause harm: catalase breaks down hydrogen peroxide, glutathione peroxidase neutralizes other peroxides, and superoxide dismutase (SOD) neutralizes superoxide. These scavenger enzymes require an adequate supply of **selenium**, **zinc** and **manganese** in order to function well – and the limit to what they can achieve is usually exceeded. Our modern lifestyle typically generates far more free radicals than the body has mechanisms for coping.

White blood cells (leukocytes) use free radicals, in a controlled environment, to kill invading bacteria and virus-infected cells. The liver also uses free radicals to detoxify harmful chemicals. Outside this regulated environment, however, free radicals destroy cellular membranes, enzymes, genetic material, and even life itself. They accelerate aging and contribute to the development of arterial disease, cancer, and cataracts. They damage collagen by creating a cross-linkage of molecules and loss of elasticity. Wrinkled skin, stiff joints and high blood pressure are often the result of this process of deterioration.

Free radicals are released in the body from overexposure to sunlight – from the breaking down or detoxification of many chemical compounds, such as petrochemicals (in drugs, artificial food colorings, smog, etc.), preservatives in processed meats (e.g., nitrates, nitrites), rancid and adulterated fats, exhaust fumes, cleaning fluids (e.g., carbon tetrachloride), the tar in tobacco smoke, chlorinated drinking water (which can form chloroform in the body), cadmium and other heavy metals – and also from radiation (X-rays, cosmic and gamma radiation, microwaves, cell phones). The more we expose ourselves to such hazards, the greater the load of uncontrolled free radicals to which we subject our bodies – and the more likely we are to exceed the ability of our immune processes to protect us from such damage.

Some everyday food substances contribute to excess free radical production if they are consumed to excess. These include polyunsaturated oils, alcohol, and sugar. Recent studies suggest that both oxidative damage and free radical production may be linked to spikes in sugar consumption. This is one reason why diabetics are at such high risk for atherosclerosis: their arteries are continually flooded with excess levels of blood sugar (glucose).

Stress and overwork also increase our risk of free radical damage. Whether the stress itself creates free radicals or whether it prevents our immune processes from handling free radicals from other sources is unknown. Either way, the result is the same. Anything you can do to relieve stress will reduce your body's risk of free radical damage: balance work with pleasure, take daily rest breaks, meditate, do something every day just for fun, be spontaneous, exercise regularly, socialize.

Pinch Test

If you would like to know how much your body has already been affected by free radicals, there is a simple test you can do. Extend your hand, palm down, in a relaxed position. Pinch the skin on the back of your hand and lift the fold upwards. Release this fold of skin and see how long it takes to pull back into position. If you are young or have minimal free radical damage, your skin will snap back immediately. Where there is considerable cross-linkage of collagen, the skin fold will slowly draw back into place, sometimes taking several seconds.

Fats and Oils

Contrary to popular myth, *saturated fats do **not** cause heart disease.* If they did, the rural populations of western countries would have died off generations ago due to their high consumption of beef, pork, bacon, eggs, sausages, lard, etc. Natural fats that are predominately saturated are extremely stable and can still provide tiny amounts of essential fatty acids.

Contrary to another popular misconception, *polyunsaturated oils do **not** prevent heart disease.* On the contrary, *they may contribute to it.* Polyunsaturated oils are chemically unstable. This is because they have multiple loose double carbon bonds in their molecular structure. When subject to heat or air, they oxidize rapidly to form harmful free radicals. The more unsaturated the oil, the more potentially hazardous it is. Oils that are predominately unsaturated include hemp, safflower, sunflower, corn, soy, wheat germ, walnut, flax, pumpkin, and cottonseed.

The most hazardous vegetable oils of all are those used by restaurants for deep frying. These oils are heated and re-heated many times over. They are rancid; however, deodorants added by the manufacturers disguise the smell of rancidity.

Other very hazardous oils are those which have been hydrogenated to form margarine, shortening or other adulterated fats. These substances are not natural foods at all and are more correctly termed "food artifacts". They contain peroxidized fats, *trans* fatty acids, and other modified fat molecules which can compromise immune processes.

Even the so called "cold" pressed oils can be harmful, due to the heat (over 200⁰ F) generated by the friction of the processing equipment. Additionally, as soon as they are exposed to air these oils degenerate rapidly; and when used for cooking, their destruction is assured.

Healthy fatty acids are crucial to our well-being. They help to form the membranes that surround every cell in the body. (Healthy cell membranes are part of our immune defences against degenerative diseases.) Fatty acids are precursors to hormone-like substances called "prostaglandins", which help to regulate gastric secretions, pancreatic functions, and the release of pituitary hormones. Fatty acids combine with glycerol to form triglycerides, which act as carriers for vitamins A, D and E and help to convert beta carotene into vitamin A.

Fatty acids are of three basic types: <u>saturated</u> (e.g., palmitic acid, stearic acid), <u>monounsaturated</u> (e.g., oleic acid), and <u>polyunsaturated</u> (e.g., linoleic, linolenic, arachidonic). All of the fats and oils we consume consist of various proportions of these three groups. For example, ghee (clarified butter) is approximately 68% saturated, 27% monounsaturated, and 5% polyunsaturated. Olive oil is approximately 13% saturated, 79% monounsaturated, and 8% polyunsaturated.

If our diets provide an adequate supply of all of the basic fatty acids, our bodies can select the best ones for the tasks that need to be accomplished on any given day. If the best ones are not available, then our bodies are forced to do the best they can with whatever is available. ***This is how the integrity of cellular membranes becomes compromised.*** Arterial cell walls require a certain percentage of oleic acid (monounsaturated) in their membranes in order to resist deterioration from free radicals. If, however, we have not consumed sufficient monounsaturates and our bodies have not also been able to de-saturate enough saturated fats to make sufficient oleic acid, then our arterial cell membranes contain too high a percentage of the unstable polyunsaturates – increasing their susceptibility to free radical damage.

There are only two essential fatty acids: linoleic acid (omega-6) and alpha-linolenic acid (omega-3). [*"Essential" means that they must be supplied from food because our bodies cannot manufacture them.*] If we have a sufficient intake of these two – and in the presence of sufficient vitamins and minerals – the body can manufacture all of the other fatty acids it needs.

The essential fatty acids we require are found in relatively high proportions in oils that are predominantly polyunsaturated. This creates for us a balancing act, because the polyunsaturates are the ones most prone to deterioration from free radicals. Fortunately, those fats and oils that are predominantly saturated or monounsaturated also contain smaller but significant amounts of essential fatty acids.

Because it is not an essential fatty acid, ***the important role of oleic acid (omega-9) in stabilizing cellular membranes has been largely overlooked***. There is a tenuous assumption that the body should be able to make all of the omega-9 it needs if its intake of omega-3 and omega-6 fats is adequate. This happens only if conditions are ideal, and they rarely are. Mediterranean countries tend to use olive oil as a dietary staple. Doing so ensures that the body has an adequate intake of oleic acid without having to convert other fatty acids. Thus, omega-9 spares the action of omega-3's and omega-6's, leaving them available for other purposes. The incidence of heart disease is significantly lower in countries where consumption of olive oil is relatively high. Not a coincidence.

Oleic acid (omega-9) is a monounsaturated fatty acid. This means that it has only one loose double carbon bond in its molecular structure, making it much more resistant to deterioration than the polyunsaturates. Oils that are high in mononunsaturates include olive, macadamia, avocado, cashew, hickory, hazelnut/filbert, pecan, and pistachio.

Fish body oils are a source of intermediate omega-3 fatty acids, the principal one of which is EPA (eicosapentaenoic acid). EPA improves the flow characteristics of blood by preventing blood cells from sticking together to form clots that might otherwise plug narrowed arteries. EPA also tends (a) to reduce serum cholesterol levels, and (b) to increase HDL cholesterol (the "good" kind). EPA is nature's anti-freeze, so to speak, that keeps fish bodies from stiffening in cold temperatures. The colder the water the fish lives in, the higher its EPA content. Most fish will do, with some of the better sources being salmon, mackerel, krill, cod, herring, haddock, trout, whitefish, oysters, and squid.

Organic flax oil is used therapeutically to treat a number of conditions. It provides approximately 57% alpha-linolenic acid (omega-3), 16% linoleic acid (omega-6), and 18% oleic acid (omega-9). Raw flaxseed oil, however, is highly susceptible to deterioration because of its 73% content of polyunsaturates. A healthier choice is flaxseed oil that has been specially processed at 40^0 C in a controlled atmosphere of nitrogen (rather than oxygen), hermetically sealed into opaque capsules, and packaged in light-resistant bottles – all of this to resist the destructive influences of oxygen and light.

Both the quantity and quality of fats and oils we consume are critical to health. If our total fat intake is too low, we do not have enough essential fatty acids to thrive and we increase our risk for degenerative diseases. If our total fat intake is too high, the body uses first the fatty acids it can most readily assimilate, leaving the less desirable and unstable ones to circulate throughout the lymphatic system contributing to tissue damage in various locations.

Nutritional Bypass Program

What you are about to read has transformed many lives and saved countless others. It is a program designed to provide your body's innate processes with the necessary tools and conditions to re-engage a healing system that can significantly improve your health and wellbeing. Over the past 30 years, this program has grown to be called, "The Nutritional Bypass".

The complete Nutritional Bypass program involves three parts, each of which is outlined more fully in the pages that follow:

1. Reducing one's exposure to harmful factors,
2. Increasing one's intake of foods that have a protective effect, and
3. Specific high potency supplements that enable the body to remove arterial plaque.

Regular physical exercise should also be included in any nutritional bypass program, because it protects the cardiovascular system and supports immune processes. It tones muscles, eases stress, stimulates internal organs, relieves depression, helps to lower cholesterol, improves lymphatic flow, and helps one to think more clearly. The best form of exercise is one which you enjoy and will cause you to sweat for at least 30 minutes, repeated three times per week. Rapid walking, cycling, aerobics, racquet sports, team sports, martial arts – anything that can raise your pulse rate to between

120 and 140 beats per minute. **Exercise, however, does _not_ reduce arterial blockages.** There have been a number of world class athletes who have dropped dead from heart attacks.

Guidelines to follow when implementing the full program:

1. Stop smoking and/or avoid second hand tobacco smoke.
2. Reduce exposure to radiation, X-rays, exhaust fumes, and industrial pollutants.
3. Drink at least 8 glasses of purified water daily. Avoid drinking or bathing in chlorinated water.
4. Use olive oil and butter as the primary dietary fats/oils. Reduce intake of polyunsaturated oils. Strictly avoid rancid fats/oils, deep fried foods, margarines, shortening, and *trans* fats.
5. Eat fish twice weekly and/or supplement with omega-3 fish body oils.
6. Restrict consumption of concentrated sugars of all kinds (sucrose, glucose, fructose, white sugar, brown sugar, raw sugar, corn syrup, maple syrup, honey, molasses, etc.).
7. Limit alcoholic beverages to two drinks per week.
8. Limit caffeine intake (coffee, tea, colas) to the equivalent of one cup of coffee or two cups of tea (preferably green tea) daily.
9. Avoid processed meats, nitrates, nitrites and other suspect food preservatives.
10. Take the Arterial Cleansing Formula.

Following the first nine recommendations above provides for a nutritional environment as close as possible to our pre-1910 ancestors, all of whom were apparently immune to heart disease. Reducing risk factors addresses only one part of the problem, however. The other part involves strengthening immune processes not only to withstand future insults, but also to clear away the arterial plaque that has been accumulating over the years. This is the purpose of the tenth item on the above list, and the subject of our next chapter.

Arterial Cleansing Formula

The human body has an incredible, innate ability to heal itself – provided we give it the raw materials it needs to do so. *Not only are we subject to more cardiovascular risks than our heart-disease-free ancestors, our bodies are less well equipped to protect against these risks.* Our dependence on agribusiness and processed foods leaves us lacking in vital nutrients required for healthy immune function. Our stressful lifestyles, prescription drugs, refined sugar, alcohol, caffeine, food artifacts (e.g., margarine), and non-nutritive substances (e.g., artificial colorings, flavorings, preservatives) significantly increase our bodies' needs for vital nutrients at a time when those nutrients are less available in our foods. Through time, *our bodies (a) have become exposed to more free radicals than ever before, and (b) have become less well equipped to deal with those free radicals.*

The good news is that we can return our bodies to the natural cardio-protective state that our ancestors enjoyed. For over 30 years, many thousands of Canadians have been doing just that – by taking the Arterial Cleansing Formula (ACF) – a high potency, broad spectrum of select nutrients that stimulate the body's innate processes both to clear away arterial plaque and to prevent its return. The ACF works by supporting these processes in the body:

1. Neutralizing free radicals before they can cause cellular damage.
2. Protecting vital tissues from oxidative damage.

3. Eliminating homocysteine.
4. Manufacturing T-cells and macrophages to destroy mutated and damaged cells before they can accumulate in the arteries.
5. Manufacturing lipoprotein lipase (LPL) to emulsify and clear away fats from artery walls.
6. Chelating calcium, other minerals, and heavy metals from artery walls.
7. Improving the flow characteristics (viscosity) of the blood.
8. Opening up collateral blood vessels around obstructions, creating new pathways for blood to reach vital tissues.
9. Dissolving blood clots.
10. Preventing arterial spasms.

Only a comprehensive, high potency formula in a very specific synergistic combination can accomplish all of the above. All other approaches to cardio-protective supplementation are fragmentary and exclude a number of vital links in the nutritional chain.

Nutrients Required

The following is list of 19 key players on the arterial cleansing team. There are 8 other nutrients required in a supportive role, to enable the body to make the most efficient use of these 19. For best results, all 27 need to be present in optimal amounts.

Vitamin A. Stimulates the thymus gland to grow in size, enabling it to produce more T-cells and antibodies. Increases utilization of selenium, an antioxidant.

Vitamin B-1. Facilitates removal of lead from tissues. Required for health of heart tissue.

Niacin. Helps the body to eliminate excess cholesterol.

Pantothenic Acid. Necessary for the production of healthy antibodies.

Vitamin B-6. Helps prevent methionine (a dietary amino acid) from breaking down into homocysteine, a toxic substance that can damage artery walls.

Vitamin B-12. Assists vitamin B-6 in eliminating homocysteine.

Folic Acid. Assists vitamins B-6 and B-12 in eliminating homocysteine.

Choline. Emulsifies fats that are released from the artery walls, keeping them in solution, preventing them from plugging up in narrowed arteries. Keeps fats in the blood from sticking together. Oxidizes or burns fats in the liver.

Vitamin C. A powerful antioxidant and chelating agent. Protects against heavy metals (e.g., lead, arsenic) and keeps them in solution to be eliminated via the urine. Stimulates the production of lipoprotein lipase (LPL), an enzyme that dissolves fats on artery walls. Facilitates the body's internal production of coenzyme Q_{10}.

Vitamin E. A fat-soluble antioxidant. Protects against free radicals – including superoxides, hydroxyl radicals, peroxides, and hydroperoxides. Dissolves clots in the bloodstream and helps to prevent their re-formation. Increases the body's ability to grow collateral blood vessels around damaged areas. Keeps blood platelets from sticking together.

Manganese. A free radical inhibitor.

Magnesium. Keeps calcium in solution, preventing it from being deposited in arterial plaque. Helps to remove calcium from arterial plaque. Helps to regulate heartbeat. Prevents arterial spasms.

Potassium. Helps to normalize blood pressure. Helps to regulate heartbeat.

Zinc. A free radical inhibitor. Helps the body to utilize vitamin A.

Selenium. 200 to 500 times more potent than vitamin E as an antioxidant. The body incorporates it into glutathione peroxidase, an antioxidant enzyme that detoxifies hydrogen peroxide and fatty acid peroxides. Assists vitamin E in inhibiting free radicals and protecting tissues from oxidative damage.

L-Cysteine Hydrochloride. An amino acid that acts as a chelating agent. Assists in the termination of free radicals produced by ionizing radiation.

DL-Methionine. A chelating agent and free radical scavenger. An amino acid that helps to detoxify the body and emulsify fats.

Thymus substance. Glandular tissue that supports thymus function, to produce T-cells that dispose of cells damaged by free radicals.

Potencies Required

Thirty years of experience indicate that in order to achieve optimal arterial cleansing it is necessary to take all of the following supplemental nutrients daily, within the ranges recommended beside each. There is no one miracle ingredient in this formula. It is this very special combination of all 27, working together and supporting each other, like instruments in an orchestra.

Vitamin A	22,000 to 40,000 I.U.
Vitamin D	40 to 65 I.U.
Vitamin C	4,000 to 4,400 mg.
Vitamin E	600 to 650 I.U.
Vitamin B-1 (thiamine)	66 to 200 mg.
Vitamin B-2 (riboflavin)	30 to 55 mg.
Vitamin B-6 (pyridoxine)	50 to 150 mg.
Vitamin B-12`	160 to 550 mcg.
Niacin	44 to 70 mg.
Niacinamide	20 to 50 mg.
Pantothenic Acid	330 to 550 mg.
Folic Acid	0.4 to 2.2 mg.
Biotin	50 to 122 mg.
Choline (bitartrate)	440 to 725 mg.
Inositol	40 to 55 mg.
DL-Methionine	160 to 550 mg.
Magnesium (oxide)	400 to 555 mg.
Potassium (chloride)	400 to 444 mg.
Manganese (gluconate)	5 to 22 mg.
Zinc (gluconate)	25 to 33 mg.
Chromium (chelated)	130 to 333 mcg.
Selenium (chelated)	200 to 330 mcg.
Betaine hydrochloride	120 to 130 mg.
L-Cysteine hydrochloride	660 to 1,000 mg.
Thymus concentrate	55 to 100 mg.
Spleen concentrate	55 to 100 mg.
Adrenal concentrate	40 to 100 mg.

Needless to say, it is not possible to fit all of the above nutrients into a single tablet that is capable of being swallowed. It is necessary either (a) to piece together many tablets/capsules of fragmentary supplements, or (b) to take 10 tablets per day of a homogeneous supplement which combines all 27 nutrients in the above proportions.

Protocol

To achieve optimal arterial cleansing it is usually necessary to take 10 homogeneous ACF tablets daily for one month for every 10 years of age (e.g., 4 months for someone aged 40, 6 months for someone aged 60, etc.) When this initial cleansing is completed, it is recommended to stay on a maintenance level of 5 tablets per day, in order to prevent the plaque from returning. Some people on this maintenance program like to bump up their intake to 10 tablets per day for a month or two every year, analogous to a "spring cleaning".

Because diabetics are at such a high risk for arterial damage it is best for them to stay on 10 tablets of the ACF daily forever. Anyone who has had a heart attack, stroke, or bypass surgery will have scarring left behind after the plaque has been removed. For this reason, they also are well advised to stay on 10 tablets per day for life. Scars tend to attract debris, thus re-initiating the buildup of arterial plaque.

The most efficient way to utilize the ACF is to take the 10 tablets per day in divided amounts with meals. This could be 3 tablets with breakfast, 4 with lunch, 3 with supper – or 5 with breakfast, 5 with supper. It is important to take the tablets with food so that the nutrients in the meal and the nutrients in the tablets support and enhance each other.

Digestive Support

Taking 10 tablets per day of the ACF should turn the urine a bright yellow color. This is caused by a tiny percentage of unused vitamin C that spills over into the urine. *Pale urine while taking the ACF indicates digestive weakness*: the tablets are not being broken down and absorbed from the digestive tract. The solution in this case is to take supplementary digestive enzymes with each meal. The most effective digestive support formula is one that includes betaine hydrochloride and bile plus a broad spectrum of protease, amylase and lipase enzymes. Take as many digestive aid tablets per meal as required to bring a bright yellow color to the urine.

Frequently Asked Questions

Does the Arterial Cleansing Formula work for everyone?

Over the last 30 years there have been approximately 25 reports where the person taking the ACF received no perceptible benefits. In most of these cases there was an underlying digestive weakness indicated by pale colored urine (i.e., not breaking down the tablets and absorbing the nutrients). In a few of these cases, the person's hyper-stressful lifestyle may have overridden any benefit that the ACF might have been able to provide. One gentleman was constantly on the go, pushed himself to do one task after the other, ate on the run, never took time to rest; EDTA chelation therapy was not able to help him either.

How long will it take to feel any results on the arterial cleansing program?

This is a variable. We are all different. Most people start to notice slight improvements in about three weeks – such as having more energy, better skin tone, and requiring less sleep. Some are able to get complete relief from their angina or leg pains in about six weeks. Optimal arterial cleansing usually takes about one month for every 10 years of age.

Are there any side effects to arterial cleansing?

Not as such. The ingredients in the formula are natural and safe. *About five percent of people,* however, *may have temporary cleansing reactions* lasting for 5 or 10 days – including headaches, nausea, indigestion, diarrhea, fatigue, or excessive intestinal gas. These are indications that the eliminative systems of the body are catching up with the release of debris from the plaque. During a cleansing reaction there are two choices: (1) reduce the number of tablets to 3 per day, then each day add one more tablet, gradually working back up to 10, or (2) continue on the 10 tablets per day knowing that the cleansing reaction will soon subside.

Will the Arterial Cleansing Formula conflict with any prescription drugs I am taking?

There is no known conflict between the nutrients in ACF and any prescription drugs, with the possible exception that some antibiotics tend to cancel out vitamin C, and vice versa – in which case taking the antibiotics two hours apart from the ACF eliminates the conflict. *If you are on prescribed medication, you need to have it monitored by your doctor.* As your body gradually improves on the ACF, you will likely require less of your prescribed drugs. Your doctor and your pharmacist are the professionals qualified to counsel you about your drugs.

I am scheduled for bypass surgery in three weeks. Should I call off the surgery and try the arterial cleansing program instead?

That is a judgment call that only you can make. It is unlikely that the ACF is able to remove significant blockages in only three weeks. If the surgery could safely be postponed for at least three months, that would give the ACF a much better opportunity to prove its worth. If you opt for the surgery, then know that the ACF will help fortify your body to go through the operation, to heal faster, to prevent plaque from recurring where the blood vessels have been sutured, and will also remove plaque in areas not accessible to the surgeon.

Will the Arterial Cleansing Formula pull away chunks of plaque that could plug up further downstream?

No. This is not how it works. The plaque is scrubbed away, safely and gradually, with a detergent-like action. There are enough emulsifiers (e.g., choline, methionine) in the ACF to keep fats in solution so that they do not plug up elsewhere.

Is it a good idea to take aspirin-like drugs during the arterial cleansing program? I have heard that aspirin helps to prevent heart attacks by making the blood thinner.

Most people do not have blood which is too "thick", but rather have blood cells which tend to clump or stick together. In addition to everything else the ACF does, it also improves the flow characteristics (or "slipperiness") of the blood, enabling it to flow more freely. Additional supplements of omega-3 fish body oils can sometimes further improve the blood's flow characteristics (viscosity).

Will the Arterial Cleansing Formula replace all of the other dietary supplements I am presently taking?

It is usually of benefit to take supplementary omega-3 fish oils in addition to the ACF. If you are taking cholesterol lowering drugs, it is also beneficial to take supplementary CoQ_{10}. If you are taking any herbal or homeopathic remedies that are working for you, by all means continue them. Unless you have an unusually high requirement for a particular vitamin or mineral, your body is not likely to need any more than those that are provided in the ACF.

I am concerned about potential toxicity from the high level of vitamin A in the Arterial Cleansing Formula.

The Merck Index (a medical school textbook) suggests that chronic toxicity may develop after taking over 100,000 I.U. of vitamin A daily over a period of months. This is from 2.5 to 4.5 times higher than the level of vitamin A in the ACF, depending on which version of this formula one is taking. In 30 years there have been zero reports of vitamin A toxicity attributed to the ACF.

Confirming Research

Research studies test hypotheses (i.e., suppositions or educated guesses) based on a particular set of assumptions. Studies cannot prove a cause and effect relationship, however. All they can do is measure a correlation between two variables that either supports or does not support the presumed hypothesis.

The Arterial Cleansing Formula does not lend itself to double blind studies. This is because vitamin C and riboflavin turn the urine a bright yellow color. Everyone participating in the study would instantly know if they were receiving the real formula or a placebo. Even if a double blind study were possible, it is not necessary. Thirty years of successes tells us that the ACF works. Time is the best test of all.

There is voluminous research supporting the use of specific single nutrients in both preventing and treating cardiovascular diseases. Listed below are references to 132 studies conducted over a 40-year period which document the effectiveness of 11 of the ingredients in the Arterial Cleansing Formula.

Vitamin E

Hennig B, Boissonneault GA. *The roles of vitamin E and oxidized lipids in atherosclerosis.* Int Clin Nutr Rev 8(3):1349, 1998.

Cockroft J, Chowiencyk P. *Beyond cholesterol reduction in coronary heart disease: Is vitamin E the answer?* Heart 76:193-4, 1996.

Jialal I, Fuller CJ. *Effect of vitamin E, vitamin C and beta-carotene on LDL oxidation and atherosclerosis.* Can J Cardiol ll(Suppl G):97G-1036, 1995.

Fuller CJet al. *Effects of increasing doses of alpha-tocopherol in providing protection of low-density lipoprotein from oxidation. AmJCardiol8l(2):231-3, 1998.*

Calzada C et al. *The influence of antioxidant nutrients on platelet function in healthy volunteers. Atherosclerosis 128(1):97-105, 1997.*

Meyer F et al. *Lower ischemic heart disease incidence and mortality among vitamin supplement users. Can J Cardiol 12:930-4, 1996.*

Rimm EB et al. *Vitamin E consumption and the risk of coronary heart disease in men. N Engl J Med 328(20):1450-6, 1993.*

Piesse JW. *Vitamin E and peripheral vascular disease. Int Clin Nutr Rev 4(4):178-82, 1984.*

Kritchevsky SB et al. *Dietary antioxidants and carotid artery wall thickness: the ARIL study. Circulation 92(8): 214250, 1995.*

Bellizi MC et al. *Vitamin E and coronary heart disease: the European paradox. Eur J Clin Nutr 48:822-31, 1994.*

Stampfer et al. *Vitamin E consumption and the risk of coronary disease in women. N EnjZl J Med 328: 1444-9, 1993.*

Carpenter KLHet al. *Depletion of alpha-tocopherol in human atherosclerotic lesions. Free Rad Res 23:549-58, 1995.*

Messetti A et al. *Vitamins E & C and lipid peroxidation in plasma and arterial tissue of smokers and nonsmokers. Atherosclerosis 112:91-9, 1995.*

Hodis HNet al. *Serial coronary angiographic evidence that antioxidant vitamin intake reduces progression of coronary artery atherosclerosis. JAMA 273(2):1849-54, 1995.*

Stephens NG et al. *Randomized controlled trial of vitamin E in patients with coronary disease. Cambridge Heart Antioxidant Study (CHAOS). Lancet 347: 781-6, 1996.*

Miwa K et al. *Vitamin E deficiency in variant angina. Circulation 94(1):14-18, 1996.*

Yau TM et al. *Vitamin E for coronary bypass operations. A prospective, double-blind, randomized trial. J Thorac Cardiovasc Sure 108(2): 302-10, 1994.*

Cavarochi NC et al. *Superoxide generation during cardiopulmonary bypass: is there a role for vitamin E? J SurQ Res 40:519-27, 1986.*

DeMaio SJet al. *Vitamin E supplementation, plasma lipids and incidence of restenosis after percutaneous transluminal coronary angioplasty (PCTA). JAm Coll Nutr 11(I):68-73, 1992.*

De Lorgeril M et al. *Beneficial effect of dietary antioxidant supplementation on platelet aggregation and cyclosporine treatment in heart transplant recipients. Transplantation 58:193-4, 1994.*

Gey KFet al. Inverse correlation between plasma vitamin E and mortality from ischemic heart disease in cross-cultural epidemiology. Am J Clin Nutr 53: 326S-34S, 1991.

Japanese Cerebrovasular Prevention Study reported in: Secondary prevention tried in pateints with cerebrovascular accident. Medical Tribune Meeting Focus Suppl, May 22, 1997:4.

Fumimoto S et al. Protective effect of vitamin E on cerebral ischemia. SurQ Neuro 22(5): 449-54, 1984.

Wen Yet al. Lipid peroxidation and antioxidant vitamins C and E in hypetensive patients. Irish JMed 165(3):210-12, 1996.

Kanofsky JD, Kanofsky PB. Prevention of thromboembolic disease by vitamin E. Letter. N Enel J Med 305(3):173-4, 1981.

Vitamin C

Chakraberry S et al. Protective role of ascorbic acid against lipid peroxidation and myocardial injury. Molec Cell Biochem 111:41-7, 1992.

Jialal 1, Grundy S. Effect of combined supplementation with alpha-tocopherol, ascorbate, and beta carotene on lowdensity lipoprotein oxidation. Circulation 88:2780-6, 1993.

Knekt P et al. Antioxidant vitamin intake and coronary mortality in a longitudinal population study. Am JEpidemiol 139:1180-9, 1994.

Manson J et al. A prospective study of vitamin C and incidence of coronary heart disease in women. Circulation 85:865, 1992.

Willis GS. The reversibility of atherosclerosis. Can Med Assoc J 77:106-10, 1957.

Nyyssonen K et al. Vitamin C deficiency and risk of myocardial infarction: prospective population study of men from Eastern Finland. BMJ 314: 634-8.

Spittle CR. Vitamin C and deep-vein thromboses. Lancet ii:199-201,1973.

Ginter E et al. Vitamin C in the control of hypercholesterolemia in man. Int J Vitam Nutr Res Suppl 23:137-52, 1982.

Turley S et al. Role of ascorbic acid in the regulation of cholesterol metabolism and the pathogenesis of atherosclerosis. Atherosclerosis 24:1-18, 1976.

Toohey L et al. Plasma ascorbic acid concentrations are related to cardiovascular risk factors in Aftrican-Americans. J Nutr 126:121-8, 1996.

Simon J. Vitamin C and cardiovascular disease: a review. J Am Coll Nutr 11:107-25, 1992.

Jacques PF et al. Effect of vitamin C supplementation in lipoprotein cholesterol, apoliprotein, and triglyceride concentration. Ann Epidemiol 5(1):52-9, 1995.

Bordie A et al. Effect of vitamin C on platelet adhesiveness and platelet aggregation in coronary artery disease patients. Clin Cardol 8(10):552-4, 1985.

Khaw K- T, Woodhouse P. *Interrelation of vitamin C, infection, hemostatic factors and cardiovascular disease. BMJ 310:1559-63, 1995.*

Bordia AK. *The effect of vitamin C on blood lipids, fibrinolytic activity and platelet adhesiveness in patients with coronary artery disease. Atherosclerosis 35:181-7, 1980.*

Levine GN. *Ascorbic acid reverses endothelial vasomotor dysfunction in patients with coronary artery disease. Circulation 93(6):1107-13, 1996.*

Dingchae H et al. *The protective effects of high-dose ascorbic acid on myocardium against reperfusion injury during and after cardiopulmonary bypass. Thorac Cardiovasc SurQ 42(5): 276-8, 1994.*

Tomoda Het al. *Possible prevention of postangioplasty restenosis by ascorbic acid. Am JCardioloQV 78(11):1284-6, 1996.*

Willis GC et al. *Serial arteriography in atherosclerosis. Can Med Assoc J 71:562-8, 1954.*

Solzbach U et al. *Vitamin C improves endothelial dysfunction of epicardial coronary arteries in hypertensive patients. Circulation 96(5):1513-9, 1997.*

Daviglus M et al. *Dietary vitamin C, Beta-carotene and 30 year risk of stroke: Results from the Western Electric Study. NeuroepidemioloQy 16(2):69-77, 1997.*

Gey KF et al. *Poor plasma status of carotene and vitamin C is associated with higher mortality from ischemic heart disease and stroke: Basel Prospective Study. Clin Invest 71:3-6, 1993.*

Rath M, Pauling I. *Solution to the puzzle of human cardiovascular disease: its primary cause in ascorbate deficiency leading to the deposition of lipoprotein(a) and fibrinogenl fibrin in the vascular wall. JOrthomol Med 6(3-4):125-34, 1991.*

McCarron DA et al. *Blood pressure and nutrient intake in the United States. Science 224(4656):1392-8, 1984.*

Ness AR et al. *Vitamin C status and blood pressure. JHypertens 14(4):503-8, 1996.*

Jacques PF. Effects of vitamin C on high-density lipoprotein cholesterol and blood pressure. JAm Coll Nutr 11(2):13944, 1992.

Osilesi O et al. *Bloodpressure and plasma lipids during ascorbic acid supplementation in borderline hypertensive and normotensive adults. Nutr Res 11:405-12, 1991.*

Ghosh S et al. *A double-blind, placebo-controlled parallel trial of vitamin C treatment in elderly patients with hypertension. GerontoloQV 40:268-72, 1994.*

Folic Acid

Boushey CJ et al. A quantitative assessment of plasma homocysteine as a risk factor for vascular disease: Probable benefits of increasing folic acid intakes. JAMA 274(13):1049-57, 1995.

Stampfer MJ Malinow MR. Can lowering homocysteine reduce cardiovascular risk? Editorial. N Engl J Med 332(5):328-9, 1995.

Rimm EB et al. Folate and vitamin B-6 from diet and supplements in relation to risk of coronary heart disease among women. JAMA 279(5):359-64, 1998.

Schwartz SM. Myocardial infarction in young women in relation to plasma total homocysteine, folate, and a common variant in the methylenetetrahvdrofolate reductase gene. Circulation 96(2): 412-7, 1997.

Oster KA. The treatment of bovine xanthine oxidase initiated atherosclerosis by folic acid. Clin Res 24:512A, 1976.

Kopjas TL. Effect of folic acid on collateral circulation in diffuse chronic arteriosclerosis. J Am Geriatr Soc 14(ll):1187-92, 1966.

Selhub J et al. Association between plasma homocysteine concentrations and extracranial carotid-artery stenosis. N Fnjzl J Med 332(5): 286-91, 1995.

lbbink J et al. Vitamin requirements for the treatment of hyperhomocysteine in humans. JNutr 124:1927-33, 1994.

Morrison Hl et al. Serum folate and risk of fatal coronary heart disease. JA MA 275:1893-6, 1996.

Vitamin B-6

Yerhoef P et al. Homocysteine metabolism and risk of myocardial infarction: relation with vitamin B-6, B- 12 and jolate. Am J Eyidemioll 43(9):845-59, 1996.

Zoler MI High folic acid intake lowers heart attack risk. every additional 100 mcg. cuts Ml risk 6%. Family Practice News August I, 1997;1.

Robinson K et al. Hyperhomocysteinemia and low pyridoxal phosphate: common and independent reversible risk factors for coronary artery disease. Circulation 92(10):2825-30, 1995.

Kuzuya F Vitamin B-6 and arteriosclerosis. NaQOVa JMed Sc 55(1-4):1-9, 1993.

Subbafao K et al. Pyridoxal 5 phosphate - a new physiological inhibitor of blood coagulation and platelet function. Biochem Pharmacol 28.531-4, 1979.

Kuzuya F. Vitamin B-6 and arteriosclerosis. NaQOVa J Med Sc 55(I-4):1-9, 1993.

Brattstrom L et al. *Pyridoxine reduces cholesterol and low-density-lipoprotein and increases antithrombin acivity in 80 year old men with low plasma pyridoxal 5 phosphate.* Scand J Clin Lab Invest 50(8):873-7, 1990

Selhub J et al. *Association between plasma homocysteine concentations and extracranial carotid-artery stenosis.* N EnQl JMed 332(5):286-91, 1995.

Ubbink JB et al. *The effect ofsubnormal vitamin B-6 status on homocysteine metabolism.* J Clin Invest 98(1):177-84, 1996.

Boers GH et al. *Heterorygosity for homocystinuria in premature peripheral and cerebral occlusive arterial disease.* N EnQl J Med 313(12): 709-I5, 1985.

Robinson K et al. *Low circulating folate and vitamin B-6 concentrations: risk factors for stroke, peripheral vascular disease, and coronary artery disease. European COMA C Group.* Circulation 97(5):437-43, 1998.

Boers GH. *Hyperhomocysteinaemia: a newly recognized risk factor for vascular disease.* Neth J Med 45(l):34-4l, 1994.

Aybak M et al. *Effect of oral pyridoxine hydrochloride supplementation on arterial blood pressure in patients with essential hypertension.* Arzneimittelforsch 45:1271-3, 1995.

Vitamin B-12

Lussier-Cacan S et al. *Plasma total homocysteine in healthy subjects: sex-specific relation with biological traits.* Am J Clin Nutr 64:587-93, 1996.

Brattstrom LE et al. *Higher total plasma homocysteine in vitamin B-l2 deficiency than in heterozygosity for homocystinuria due to cystathione beta-synthase deficiency.* Metabolism 37(2):175-8, 1988.

Clarke R et al. *Hyperhomocysteinemia: an independent risk factor for vascular disease.* N Enpl J Med 324(17):114955, 1991.

Calcium

Denke M et al. *Short-term dietarv calcium fortification increases focal saturated fat content and reduces serum lipids in men.* J Nutr 123:1047-53, 1993.

McCarron DA. *Is calcium more important than sodium in the pathogenesis of essential hypertension?* Hypertension 7(4):607-27, 1985.

Harlan WK et al. *Blood pressure and nutrition in adults. The National Health and Nutrition Examination Survey.* Am J Epidemiol 120:17-24, 1984.

Quereda C. *Urinary calcium excretion in treated and untreated essential hypertension.* JAm Soc Neyhrol 7(7):1058-65, 1996

Hvarfner A et al. *Indices of mineral metabolism in relation to blood pressure in a sample of a healthy population.* Acta Med Scand 219(5): 461-8, 1986.

Resnick LM. *Alterations of dietary calcium intake as a therapeutic modality inessential hypertension.* <u>Can J Physiol Pharmcaol</u>64(6):803-7, 1986.

Bucher et al. *Effects of dietary calcium supplementation on blood pressure: a meta-analysis of randomized controlled trials.* <u>JAMA</u> 275:1016-22, 1996.

Allender P et al. *Dietary calcium and blood pressure: a meta-analysis of randomized clinical trials.* <u>Ann Intern Med</u> 124:825-31, 1996.

Magnesium

Ma Jet al. *Associations of serum and dietary magnesium with cardiovascular disease, hypertension, diabetes, insulin and carotid artery wall thickness: the ARIC study.* <u>J Clin Epidemiol</u> 48(7): 927-40, 1995.

Rasmussen HS et al. *Magnesium deficiency inpatients with ischemic heart disease with and without acute myocardial infarction uncovered by intravenous loading test.* <u>Arch Intern Med</u> 148:329-32, 1988.

Satake X et al. *Relation between severity of magnesium deficiency and frequency of anginal attacks in men with variant angina.* <u>JAm Coll Cardiol</u> 28:897-902, 1996.

Igawa A et al. *Comparison of frequency of magnesium deficiency inpatients with vasospastic and fixed coronary artery disease.* <u>Am JCardiol</u>75:728-31, 1995.

Gawaz M. *(Antithrombocytic effectiveness of magnesium.]* <u>Fortschr Med</u> 114: 329-32, 1996.

Gartside PS Glueck CJ. *The important role of modifiable dietary and behavioral characteristics in the causation and prevention of coronary heart disease hospitalization and mortality: the prospective NHANES I follow-up study.* <u>J Am</u> <u>Coll Nutr</u> 14(1):71-9, 1995.

Howard JMH *Magnesium deficiency in peripheral vascular disease.* <u>J Nutr Med</u> 1:39-49, 1990.

Neglen P et al. *Peroral magnesium hydroxide therapy and intermittent claudication.* Vasa 14(3):285-8, 1985.

Dychner T, Wester PO. *Magnesium and potassium in serum and muscle in relation to disturbances of cardiac rhythm, in* <u>Magnesium, Health and Disease</u>. Spectrum Publishing Company, 1980:551-7.

Nebrand C et al. *Cardiovascular mortality and morbidity in seven counties in Sweden in relation to water hardness and geological settings.* <u>Eur Heart J</u> 13:721-7, 1992.

Yang CY. *Calcium and magnesium in drinking water and risk of death from cerebrovascular disease.* <u>Stroke</u> 29(2): 41114, 1998.

Fehlinger R et al. *Hypomagnesemia and transient ischemic cerebral attacks.* <u>Magnesium Bull</u> 6:100-4, 1984.

Gartside PS, Glueck CJ. *The important role of modifiable dietary and behavioral characteristics in the causation and prevention of coronary heart disease hospitalization and mortality: the prospective NHANES I follow-up study.* J.Am Coll Nutr 14(1):71-9, 1995.

Altura BT Altura BM. *Interactions of Mg and K on cerebral vessels --aspects in view of stroke. Review of present status and new findings.* Magnesium 3(4-6):195-211, 1984.

Altura BM, Altura BT. *Magnesium ions and contraction of vascular smooth muscles: relationship to some vascular diseases.* Fed Proc 40(12):2672-9, 1981.

Seeling M Set al. *Low magnesium: a common denominator in pathologic processes in diabetes mellitus, cardiovascular disease and eclampsia. Abstract.* JAm Coll Nutr 11(5):597-637, 1992.

Hatton D et al. *Mechanisms of calcium's effects on blood pressure.* Semin Nephrol 15:593-602, 1995.

Joffres MR et al. *Relationship of magnesium intake and other dietary factors to blood pressure: the Honolulu heart study.* Am JClin Nutr 45(2):469-75, 1987.

Fischer PWFet al. *Magnesium status and excretion in age-matched subjects with normal and elevated blood pressures.* Clin Biochem 26:207-11, 1993.

Seeling MS et al. *Low magnesium: a common denominator in pathologic processes in diabetes melitus, cardiovascular disease and eclampsia. Abstract.* JAm Coll Nutr 11(5):597-637, 1992.

Kisters K et al. *Plasma magnesium and total intracellular magnesium ion content of lymphocytes in untreated normotensive and hypertensive patients.* Trace Elem Electrolytes 13(4):163-6, 1996.

Resnick L Metal. *Intracellular free magnesium in erythrocytes of essential hypertension: Relationship to blood pressure and serum divalent cations.* Proc Natl Acad Sci USA 81(2): 6511-5, 1984.

Sanjuliani AF et al. *Effects of magnesium on blood pressure and intracellular ion levels of Brazilian hypertensive patients.* Int J Cardiol 56:177-83, 1996.

Witteman JCM et al. *Reduction of blood pressure with oral magnesium supplementation in women with mild to moderate hypertension.* Am JClin Nutr 60.129-35, 1994.

Reusser M, McCarron D. *Micronutrient effects on blood pressure regulation.* Nutr Rev 52:367-75, 1994.

Witteman et al. *A prospective study of nutritional factors and hypertension among US women.* Circulation 80.: 1320-7, 1989.

Altura BM, Altura BT. *Interactions of Mg and K on blood vessels: Aspects in view of hypertension.* <u>Magnesium</u> 3(46):175-94, 1984.

Potassium

Young DB et al. *Potassium's cardiovascular protective mechanisms.* <u>Am J Physiol</u> 268(4 Pt 2): 8825-8837, 1995.

Singh RB et al. *Effect of treatment with magnesium and potassium on mortality and reinfarction rate* of *patients with suspected acute myocardial infarction.* <u>Int J Clin Pharmacol Ther</u> 34:219-25, 1996.

Khaw KT, Barrett-Connor E. *Dietary potassium and stroke-associated mortality. A 12 year prospective population study.* <u>N Engl J Med</u> 316(5):235-40, 1987.

Luft F Weinberger M. *Potassium and blood pressure regulation.* <u>Am J Clin Nutr</u> 45:1289-94, 1987.

Gariballa SE et al. *Serum potassium following stroke.* <u>Age AQinQ</u> 24(Suppl 2):20, 1995.

Sasaki S et al. *Dietary sodium, potassium, saturated fat, alcohol, and stroke mortality.* <u>Stroke</u> 26(5): 783-9, 1995.

Gelijnse JM et al. *Sodium and potassium intake and blood pressure damage in childhood.* <u>Br Med J</u> 300:899-902, 1990.

Reusser M, McCarron D. *Micronutrient effects on blood pressure regulation.* <u>Nutr Rev</u> 52:367-75, 1994.

Barri Y, Wingo C. *The effects* of *potassium depletion and supplementation on blood pressure: a clinical review.* <u>Am J Med Sci</u> 314:37-40, 1997.

Whelton et al. *Effects of oral potassium on blood pressure: meta-analysis of randomized controlled trials.* <u>JAMA</u> 277:1624-32, 1997.

Kotchen T, Kotchen J *Dietary sodium and blood pressure interactions with other nutrients.* <u>Am JClin Nutr</u> 65: 708S11S, 1997.

Stein, P, Black H. *The role of diet in the genesis and treatment of hypertension.* <u>Med Clin N Am</u> 77:831-47, 1993.

Khaw KT, Barrett-Connor E. *The association between blood pressure, age, and dietary sodium and potassium. A population study.* <u>Circulation</u> 77(1):53-61, 1998.

Suter P. *Potassium and hypertension.* <u>Nutr Rev</u> 56(5): 151-3, 1998.

Smith WCS et al. *Urinary electrolyte excretion, alcohol consumption, and blood pressure in the Scottish heart study.* <u>Br Med J</u> 297: 329-30, 1998.

Krishna GG. *Role of potassium in the pathogenesis of hypertension.* <u>Am J Med Sci</u> 307 Suppl 1: S21-5, 1994.

Trevisian M et al. *Red blood cell sodium and potassium concentration and blood pressure.* <u>Ann Epidemiol</u> 5:44-51, 1994.

Capuccio FP *et al. Does potassium supplementation lower blood pressure? A meta-analysis of published trials. J Hypertens 9.465-73, 1991.*

Whelton PK *et al. Effects of oral potassium on blood pressure. Meta-analysis of randomized controlled clinical trials. JAMA 277(20):1624-32, 1997.*

Chromium

Simonoff M. *Chromium deficiency and cardiovascular risk. Cardiovasc Res 18(10):591-6, 1984.*

F'lad M et al. Concentration of copper, zinc, chromium, iron and nickel in the abdominal aorta of patients deceased with coronarv heart disease. J Trace Elem Electrolytes Health Dis 8(2):111-14, 1994.

Simonoff Met al. Low plasma chromium in patients with coronary artery and heart disease. Biol Trace Element Res 6:431, 1984.

Selenium

Mihailovic MB *et al. Blood and plasma selenium levels and GSH-Px activities in patients with arterial hypertension and chronic heart disease. JEnviron Pathol Toxicol Oncol 17(3-4):285-9, 1998.*

Salonen JT et al. Blood pressure, dietary fats, and antioxidants. Am J Clin Nutr 48:1226-32, 1998.

Zinc

Gatto LM, Samman S. *The effect of zinc supplementation on plasma lipids and low-density lipoprotein oxidation in males. Free Rad Biol Med 19(4):517-21, 1995.*

Singal PK *et al. Protective action of zinc against catecholamine-induced myocardial changes. Electrocardiographic and ultrastructural studies. Lab Invest 44:426, 1981.*

Fortes C *et al. Zinc supplementation and plasma lipid peroxides in an elderly population. Eur J Clin Nutr 5l (2): 97101, 1997.*